Kaplan Radiography Exam

Third Edition

Kaplan Radiography Exam

Third Edition

Karen Bonsignore, MA, RT
Myke Kudlas, MEd, RT
Dana Maiellaro, MEd, RT
Abraham Thengampallil, MD
Stinsey S. Thengampallil, RT

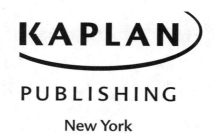

PUBLISHING

New York

This publication is designed to provide accurate and authoritative information in regard to the subject matter covered. It is sold with the understanding that the publisher is not engaged in rendering legal, accounting, or other professional service. If legal advice or other expert assistance is required, the services of a competent professional should be sought.

© 2011 by Kaplan, Inc.

Published by Kaplan Publishing, a division of Kaplan, Inc.
395 Hudson Street, 4th Floor
New York, NY 10014

Printed in the United States of America

10 9 8 7 6 5 4 3 2 1

ISBN 13: 978-1-60714-837-1

AVAILABLE ONLINE

Free Additional Practice

kaptest.com/booksonline

As owner of this book, you are entitled to additional practice online. Log on to kaptest.com/booksonline to access a full-length practice test.

Access to this material is free of charge to purchasers of this book. You will be asked for a specific password from the text in this book, so have your book handy when you log on.

For Any Test Changes or Late-Breaking Developments

kaptest.com/publishing

The material in this book is up to date at the time of publicatoin. However, the ARRT™ may have instituted changes in the test after this book was published. Be sure to carefully read the material you receive when you register for the test. If there are any important late-breaking developments— or any changes or corrections to the Kaplan test preparation materials in this book—we will post that information online at kaptest.com/publishing.

Feedback and Comments

kaplansurveys.com/books

We'd love to hear your comments and suggestions about this book. We invite you to fill out our online survey form at kaplansurveys.com/books. Your feedback is extremely valuable as we continue to develop high-quality resources to meet your needs.

Table of Contents

About the Authors

Karen Bonsignore, MA, RT(R)(M)(MR)(QM)(CT)

(Patient Care and Education) ("Extremities" in Radiographic Procedures)

Karen Bonsignore is an associate professor in the Department of Radiologic Technology and Medical Imaging at New York City College of Technology and is currently the project director of the Career ePortfolio web design project. She is certified in advanced imaging modalities, including mammography, quality management, and magnetic resonance imaging and computerized tomography. She has given numerous presentations on various radiology topics, most extensively mammography and breast imaging.

Myke Kudlas, MEd, RT(R)(QM)

(Image Production and Evaluation) (Equipment Operation and Quality Control)

Myke Kudlas is the director of the Mayo Clinic Radiography Program in Jacksonville, Florida, and assistant professor of Radiology in the Mayo Clinic College of Medicine. He has written and presented extensively in the areas of radiography and education, and is an active member of the American Society of Radiologic Technologists, the Association of Educators in Imaging and Radiologic Sciences, and the Jacksonville Society of Radiologic Technologists. He is a former item writer for the Developmental Testing Program of the College of St. Catherine and the American Registry of Radiologic Technologists.

Dana Maiellaro, MEd, RT(R)(M)

(Radiographic Procedures)

Dana Maiellaro is an instructor in the Radiologic Technology Program at Nassau Community College. She also has an advanced certification in mammography. She has been program director of the Robert J. Hochstim School of Radiography at South Nassau Communities Hospital in New York and an assistant professor in the Department of Radiologic Technology and Medical Imaging at New York City College of Technology. Her area of expertise is radiographic positioning and procedures, which she obtained working as both a diagnostic radiographer and CT technologist at several Level 1 trauma centers.

Abraham Thengampallil, MD

(Overview of the Test; Testing, Exam Style; Tackling the Computer-Based Test (CBT); The Licensure Process)

Until recently, Dr. Abraham Thengampallil was associate director of Medical Curriculum for Kaplan Medical. He received his MD at the State University of New York Health Science Center at Brooklyn (SUNY Downstate Medical Center) and did residency training in Pediatrics at the Cincinnati Children's Hospital Medical Center. Dr. Thengampallil currently works as a medical director for a medical education/strategic communications agency in New York.

Stinsey S. Thengampallil, RT(R)

(Radiation Protection)

Stinsey S. Thengampallil has worked as a radiologic technologist in New York for more than 7 years. Her areas of clinical interest include mammography, bone densitometry, and diagnostic radiography.

She received her Associate degree in Radiologic Technology and Medical Imaging from New York City College of Technology. She is a New York state–licensed radiologic technologist certified in diagnostic radiography by the American Registry of Radiologic Technologists (ARRT). She is an active member of numerous professional organizations.

How to Use This Book

This book is not intended to replace standard textbooks in radiography. Rather, it should serve as a primary review tool in the weeks and months prior to taking the American Registry of Radiologic Technologists (ARRT) exam. Since it is not practical to re-read textbooks, you will need a resource that will provide concise, focused review. This book fills that need. It is divided into sections that correspond to the content areas represented on the registry. In this way, the student will become acclimated to the contextual layout of the exam.

The practice test in this book should be taken prior to beginning your study period—use the results to identify areas of strength and weakness and then tailor an individualized study plan. For example, if your score in Patient Care was below average, plan to spend some additional days studying this subject. Likewise, if Radiation Protection was the area in which you scored the highest, you may want to leave this section for last.

Kaplan suggests that areas in which you feel weakest should be studied first; in this way, you can spend additional review time on difficult concepts. Both practice tests should be taken in quiet areas—dedicate 3.5 hours for each test.

It is advisable to take the practice exam at a library and to limit distractions. The goal is to simulate exam-like conditions and obtain data that will help structure an effective study plan.

As you work through the items, pay particular attention to the explanations. Often, studying the explanations is a valuable study resource. Notice that for difficult questions explanations have been provided that explain the reasoning for *not* choosing the incorrect answer choices. Use this information to understand the rationale behind eliminating each distracter.

Finally, take the online practice test about a week prior to your exam date. Test 2 should be taken once the majority of your study has been completed. Use the score breakdown to fine-tune any remaining areas of weakness.

Accessing Your Online Practice Test

There is a second full-length practice test available online at www.kaptest.com/booksonline. You will be asked for a password from the text in this book, so have your book handy when you log on.

PART ONE

Preparing for the ARRT Radiography Exam

Chapter 1: **Overview of the Test**

For many student radiographers, the American Registry of Radiologic Technologists (ARRT) national certification examination in Radiography is the culmination of two years of arduous study. Students are eligible to take the exam upon completion of required didactic and clinical coursework at an accredited institution. Upon completion of the exam, student radiographers become certified by the ARRT. Radiographers must then apply for licensure in the state in which they intend to practice.

The ARRT exam, or "Registry," is a 3.5-hour exam that contains 220 multiple-choice questions. Of the 220 items, 20 are experimental or pilot questions—thus, only 200 count toward the final score. The exam is a computer-based test (CBT) that is administered at test centers across the nation. The ARRT administers a number of certification exams including: mammography, sonography, radiation therapy, magnetic resonance imaging, and nuclear medicine technology. These exams are also administered in a CBT format.

CONTENT AREAS

While the exam itself is divided into five distinct content areas, the questions are presented in a randomized fashion. The content areas tested on the exam include: Imaging Procedures; Image Acquisition and Evaluation; Radiation Protection; Equipment Operation and Quality Control; and Patient Care and Education. The number of questions per content area is specified in the table below.

Content Area	Number of Questions	Percent of Exam
Imaging Procedures	58	29.0%
Image Acquisition and Evaluation	45	22.5%
Radiation Protection	45	22.5%
Equipment Operation and Quality Control	22	11.0%
Patient Care and Education	30	15.0%

Detailed descriptions of the concepts tested in each of the five content areas can be found on the ARRT website. All of the 220 exam questions are presented in a multiple-choice format.

You will be able to use either the mouse or keyboard to select the correct answer. A significant number of questions contain images (radiographs, drawings, etc.). In addition, some items will require calculations. Examinees will be provided with calculators prior to the start of the exam.

Because the Registry is the first CBT for most examinees, there is a considerable amount of anxiety associated with this exam. The ARRT provides a tutorial that examinees can take before the start of the test. Since the computer-based testing interface is intuitive, there is no practice software available for use prior to the exam date.

The content specifications of the Registry are analyzed and modified at regular intervals. Questions are written by heath care professionals, including radiologic technologists, educators, physicians, and other allied health care workers. Existing items are periodically updated or replaced. The ARRT publishes an annual report that provides information about examinee performance. In addition, many radiography programs are provided performance profiles of their graduates. In this way schools can assess performance and modify curriculum.

SCORING

Because there are multiple versions of the Registry, all of which may vary in difficulty, a scaled score is provided by the ARRT. *A scaled score of 75 is considered a passing mark on any of the ARRT exams.* This will account for any variation in exam difficulty and testing conditions. The *cut score*, or pass–fail demarcation, is preset by the ARRT.

Essentially, a student radiographer must correctly answer about 67 percent of the items on the Registry. Scaled scores for each section (content area) of the exam are also provided; these are considered less reliable inasmuch as the number of items per section is considerably lower than total items.

What If I Fail?

Failing the Registry can be a traumatic experience. If you do receive a failing grade, do not panic. Although feelings of fear and disappointment are common after such an event, keep in mind that you have put tremendous effort into your career thus far.

The first step should be to reevaluate your study plan. Are there any specific areas of weakness you neglected? Which content area may need an extra few days of study? Did you complete all of the practice questions in this book?

Once the study plan has been determined, begin to focus on your goal. The ARRT exam in radiography can be taken up to three times after an initial failed attempt. If a student fails more than three times, he or she will have to perform some remedial education.

USING A STUDY SCHEDULE

Preparing for the Registry can be a daunting task. Most students struggle with the prospect of reviewing two years' worth of material in four weeks. However, the Registry requires a review of the fundamental principles of diagnostic radiography—*not* that you re-read your textbooks. Nonetheless, selecting the relevant information can be quite intimidating. Fortunately, only the most high-yield material is included in this book. By studying the high-yield notes and completing the practice questions, you will master the concepts most commonly tested on the Registry.

Most student radiographers have about one month of dedicated study prior to the Registry. The following study schedules are based on a one-month study period. Weekends are study breaks, and there are 19 total study days. Of course, the plan may be modified to include weekends. A full-length practice exam (Practice Test 1) is scheduled for the first day of study—this will serve as a benchmark and indicate areas of strength and weakness. Next, the schedule is divided by individual subject area. The proportionate number of days spent with each content area should correspond to its relative importance on the exam.

Notice that you should do numerous practice questions each day. Keep in mind that while 50 questions may take only an hour to complete, reviewing 50 items may take longer. But remember, reviewing explanations is an invaluable study tool. The second practice test should be taken about a week before your exam date. This will provide feedback for the final review period.

Finally, the last four days before the exam should be used to review all pertinent material. In this manner, you can consolidate all of the highest yield information. Try not to learn much new information in the few days before the exam.

The following schedule is a model for working with this review book. Feel free to adjust it to suit your needs.

Sample Study Schedule

MON	TUE	WED	THU	FRI
Take Kaplan Full-length Practice Test	Imaging Procedures	Imaging Procedures	Imaging Procedures	Imaging Procedures
	58 Questions	58 Questions	58 Questions	58 Questions
MON	**TUE**	**WED**	**THU**	**FRI**
Image Acquisition and Evaluation	Image Acquisition and Evaluation	Image Acquisition and Evaluation	Radiation Protection	Radiation Protection
45 Questions	45 Questions	45 Questions	45 Questions	45 Questions
MON	**TUE**	**WED**	**THU**	**FRI**
Equipment Operation and Quality Control	Equipment Operation and Quality Control	Patient Care and Education	Patient Care and Education	Take Kaplan Full-length Practice Test online
22 Questions	22 Questions	30 Questions	30 Questions	
MON	**TUE**	**WED**	**THU**	**FRI**
Imaging Procedures	Image Acquisition and Evaluation	Radiation Protection	Equipment Operation and Quality Control AND Patient Care and Education	EXAM DAY
REVIEW DAY	REVIEW DAY	REVIEW DAY	REVIEW DAY	
		Visit Testing Center		

Chapter 2: **Testing, Exam Style**

Standardized exams are a source of anxiety and stress for most students. Similarly, the Registry can be a stressful experience for many student radiographers. This section will provide test-taking strategies as well as specific study techniques and tips that will help you succeed on the ARRT examination.

STRATEGIES TO HELP YOU ACE THE EXAM

All of the questions you will encounter on the Registry are in a multiple-choice format, and for each item there is only one correct answer. One simple but effective strategy is to develop a standardized approach. By approaching each question in a predetermined, standardized fashion, you will free your mind to think about other things pertaining to the question.

Everyone has established personal rituals, such as brushing your teeth, showering, and drinking a cup of coffee before leaving for class in the morning. In fact, these actions are so habitual that you may not even have to consciously think of each one before performing it.

Basically, with any habit, the brain attempts to reduce conscious effort by reducing the complexity of situations. The sequence of events and complex actions are stored in your memory. Once the brain has become acclimated to such events, complex actions like brushing your teeth become almost automatic. This creates an "auto-pilot" mode that enables you to simultaneously perform mundane tasks and think about more important issues.

This should be applied to testing as well—your approach to questions should become habitual. In this way your brain is able to focus on more pertinent details while answering each question.

The following steps should be used with each question:

Step 1
Carefully *read the question* and *identify* any potential clues.

Step 2
Understand what is being asked.

Step 3
Before looking at the answer choices, put the clues together with what you are being asked and *form an answer*.

Step 4
Look at the choices. If one fits your answer, *choose* it.

Step 5
If none of the answers seem to be a good fit, use general knowledge, *decision rules*, and logic to eliminate choices.

Step 6
Select an answer choice. Remember that there is no penalty for guessing, so do not leave any questions blank.

Use the following question to practice developing a standardized approach to questions.

A technician arrives to replace a nonfunctioning X-ray tube. It is determined that the thermionic diode needs replacement. Which of the following materials comprises the filament cathode?

(A) Aluminum

(B) Copper

(C) Rhodium

(D) Tungsten

First, read the question and pay careful attention to any potential clues. The question is about the *thermionic diode* of the X-ray tube.

Next, make sure you understand what you're being asked. Essentially, the question is testing your knowledge of the components of the filament cathode. The X-ray tube is comprised of a cathode and an anode. Each is comprised of *tungsten*. The cathode is negatively charged, while the anode has a positive charge. So tungsten is a component of the filament cathode.

Finally, look at the choices and determine if any one fits your answer. In this case, (D) is tungsten.

For this question, you should have been able to determine the answer by applying Steps 1 through 4 of the standardized method to answer multiple-choice questions.

Remember, if none of the answers seems to be a good fit, use general knowledge, decision rules, and logic to eliminate choices. If you couldn't remember that tungsten was a component of the filament cathode, for instance, you still had a chance to answer correctly.

Use logic to eliminate the other choices: For example, the anode may be comprised of a copper (B) block. Also, a rotating anode may contain rhenium and rhodium (C). Thus, we can eliminate choices (B) and (C). This leaves only choices (A) and (D). Try again to eliminate one of the choices. If that is not possible, pick a choice, mark it, and move on. Never leave a question unanswered!

OTHER STRATEGIES

In addition to a standardized approach to questions, there are a number of strategies you can employ to succeed on the ARRT examination.

The 75/25 Rule

Unlike traditional multiple-choice questions, ARRT questions should be approached by reading and analyzing the vignette and question stem first and trying to predict what the answer will be. Plan to spend 75 percent of your time analyzing the scenario presented in the question. Then look at the answer choices and pick out your predicted answer. Thus, the remaining 25 percent of your time should be spent on the question. This technique will prevent distraction from the incorrect choices. The Registry is designed so that each wrong answer is within the realm of possibility. Analyze the question first and determine what is really being asked.

Clustering Questions

Doing questions in clusters or groups helps you build your concentration and stamina for test day. Students often put off doing questions until too close to the exam, or do a single item and then look at the answer. Unfortunately, you will not have this luxury on exam day. As test day approaches, you should do timed questions so you'll be comfortable answering them within the time frame of the actual exam.

Use the online practice test as a mock exam before you sit for the Registry. That way, you will get a feel for the time constraint of the exam. Additionally, it will build your mental and physical stamina.

Paraphrase the Question

Another technique that will yield examination success is paraphrasing. Simplify complicated questions by paraphrasing. You may limit the use of this technique for more complicated questions that involve patient scenarios.

Remember, most questions are designed to test basic concepts, but the test maker may try to confuse examinees with wordy patient scenarios or vignettes. Do not panic; simply rephrase the question to determine what is really being asked. Then use a standardized approach to tackle the question.

Questions with Images

Many questions include images, particularly those in the Imaging Procedures and Image Acquisition and Evaluation sections.

Unfortunately, most test-takers become anxious when they see a question with an image. The key is to use the image to help you answer the question.

The first thing to do when working with a question that contains an image is to orient yourself. Next, identify the type of study, position, and technique. Finally, recall any other information that is pertinent to the image. Often, this will provide the necessary information to answer the question.

Use the following question to practice working with images.

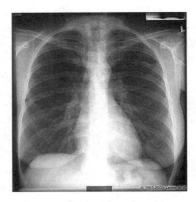

Which of the following conditions is the radiograph above used to evaluate?

1. Foreign bodies in the airway
2. Pulmonary consolidation
3. Polypoid lesions of the gastrointestinal tract

(A) 1 only

(B) 2 only

(C) 1 and 2 only

(D) 2 and 3 only

The first step should be to evaluate the image. Orient yourself by identifying the left and right side of the radiograph.

Next, identify the type of study, position, and technique. This is a PA film of the chest. The breast shadows indicate that the patient is a female.

Finally, recall any other information that is pertinent to the image that is shown. A routine chest film is taken in the PA projection in which the patient stands and faces the film cassette. The beam passes through from posterior to anterior.

Now tackle the question. Essentially, this question is asking the purpose of obtaining a PA film of the chest. Chest films are used as the primary method to evaluate the heart and lungs. Thus, this radiograph would be useful to evaluate *pulmonary pathology* (like consolidation or pneumothoraces) and to *identify the presence of foreign bodies*.

Now, look at the answer choices. This chest X-ray can be used to evaluate both foreign bodies in the airway and pulmonary consolidation. However, polypoid lesions of the gastrointestinal tract are best evaluated with a double contrast barium enema. Therefore, the correct answer is choice (C) 1 and 2 only.

COMMON PITFALLS

In addition to employing the strategies described in this chapter, you should also analyze error patterns. Most students routinely assess *overall score* and items *answered incorrectly*; while this is helpful, a more detailed analysis of specific error patterns may prove even more beneficial.

Certainly, it is worthwhile to analyze overall performance. After all, the objective of the Registry is to obtain an overall passing score. The first course of action after taking a practice test should be to calculate an overall score. You must earn a *total scaled score of 75 to pass* the Registry.

Next, review each of the five sections of the exam. What was your weakest area? Use this information to tailor a review plan; begin study with a review of your weakest subject. By focusing on areas of weakness you will maximize efficiency. This will also afford you the opportunity to study areas that you tend to avoid. Remember, spending valuable time on areas at which you excel will not increase your score.

Continue to hone in on areas of weakness while progressing through the remainder of this book. For example, if while practicing questions on Radiation Protection you realize that radiation biology is particularly difficult, spend additional time reviewing this subtopic. In this way, you will pinpoint specific areas.

The following section outlines the most common error patterns: difficulties with different question formats, anxiety, fatigue, misreading questions, emotional biases, point of view, changing answers that were already correct, and knowledge gaps.

Challenging Question Formats

The ARRT examination contains several question formats. The most common is the single-answer, traditional multiple-choice question. Also present are questions with images and items that contain numbered options that correspond to choices (A) through (D). The latter type can frustrate even the most confident student, as it requires multiple steps of reasoning.

Here is an example of such a question.

Which of the following factors can result in diminished radiograph quality?

1. Vacuum deterioration in the X-ray tube
2. Presence of air in the X-ray tube
3. Oxidation of the cathode filament

(A) 1 and 2 only

(B) 1 and 3 only

(C) 2 and 3 only

(D) 1, 2, and 3

Many student radiographers become frustrated with such questions. Although these items are not necessarily more difficult than standard multiple-choice questions, they do require multiple steps of reasoning. The most effective way to approach these items should employ the standard approach to questions, as well as paraphrasing and the 75/25 rule.

First, read the question and understand what is being asked. Basically, the exam writers are testing the student radiographer's knowledge of the factors that diminish the quality of radiographs.

Next, form an answer *before* you look at the answer choices. Remember that the vacuum in the X-ray tube provides a clear path for the electron stream. Vacuum deterioration can lead to the presence of air in the tube—this results in increased resistance and poor image quality. Air may also lead to damage (oxidation) of the X-ray tube.

The next step is to look at the numbered choices and determine which ones correspond to your predicted answer. Both vacuum deterioration and the presence of air in the X-ray tube can lead to a decrease in quality of the radiograph. Option 3, oxidation of the cathode filament, is a result of air in the X-ray tube; thus, this can also lead to a reduction in film quality. Therefore, all three options are true statements.

Finally, choose the answer choice that corresponds to your predicted answer. The correct answer is (D) because it is the only option that contains all three of the choices. Practice using this approach with all items that contain numbered options.

Anxiety and Fatigue

Anxiety is a physiologic process; it is common to feel nervous during an examination. In fact, a minimal level of anxiety can actually improve levels of alertness. However, some test-takers may suffer from debilitating anxiety that can prevent completion of an exam.

Often, errors that occur during the early stages of an exam are the result of anxiety. Adequate preparation, breathing techniques, and avoidance of caffeine can serve to decrease anxiousness.

As you practice with the questions in this book, try to monitor your own level of anxiety. If you notice that a particular question or topic tends to make you more nervous, try the following technique.

Close your eyes, lean back, and slowly rotate your neck and roll your shoulders to relax them. Take several slow, deep breaths and exhale slowly after each breath. This "mental vacation" will interrupt the feelings of anxiety and can improve concentration.

Fatigue is another common cause of errors during exams. The Registry is a 3.5-hour exam—many test-takers will find that they become tired after such a lengthy exam. You may tend to rush through the later parts of the exam because of mental and physical exhaustion. An effective method to combat fatigue is to increase stamina. Mental stamina can be increased by taking the practice tests in this book in a timed setting. Also, do questions in clusters to get a sense of how long each question should take. Physical stamina is also improved with each practice test. In addition, be sure to get enough sleep before the exam, and avoid foods that may provide a momentary burst of energy but ultimately lead to increased fatigue (junk food, candy, caffeine). Proper rest, proper diet, and effective use of practice tests can limit the effects of fatigue.

Misreading Questions

Although it is important to move through each question on the Registry in a fairly rapid manner, this can result in errors that are a product of misreading. In fact, reading mistakes are quite common during exams.

These errors may be the result of rushing or fatigue. The simple misinterpretation of a key phrase can result in an incorrect answer choice. The most effective technique to avoid such errors is to employ the 75/25 rule. Spend 75 percent of your time reading, paraphrasing, and analyzing the vignette and question stem—this will reduce errors related to misreading. By spending more time on the question itself you will identify all pertinent information. Students often miss key information by hastily reading the question and spending the majority of time on the answer choices.

Emotional Biases

Difficult exam questions can be frustrating. Identifying the types of questions that upset or frustrate you is a key component of exam readiness. As you practice with questions, identify those that you felt were too picky or any you perceived to be "trick questions." Working with such items can cause frustration; emotions can interfere with concentration and attention during an exam. Identifying such questions can help reduce errors that would normally result from emotional distraction.

Point of View

Often, exam writers change the perspective of the question to confuse students. Questions can be presented from the perspective of patients, radiographers, or other health care workers. Keep in mind that every item is designed to test a radiography concept—regardless of the point of view of the question. It is critical to identify the concept being tested and then use a standardized approach to answer the question. Use the following question to practice these concepts.

A 38-year-old construction worker who does heavy lifting arrives for a pre-employment exam. He requests a lumbar spine X-ray to evaluate his spine. The radiologist determines that the situation does not warrant this study. Which of the following is an example of an unnecessary radiographic exam?

(A) A 55-year-old male receives a chest X-ray as part of a routine physical.

(B) A 27-year-old male receives a chest X-ray as a mass screening measure for tuberculosis.

(C) An 18-year-old male receives a chest X-ray upon admission to the hospital.

(D) All of the above

This question is presented from the perspective of the patient. Don't be fooled by this—no matter what the point of view, every question must test a radiographic principle. The first step should be to read the question. Because this is a complicated scenario, try to paraphrase the question. This will streamline the question and help identify key pieces of information.

Here is the paraphrased question:

> A lumbar spine X-ray is NOT a part of a routine pre-employment exam. What are other examples of unnecessary radiographic studies?

So, basically, the objective is to choose the studies that would be deemed unnecessary. Now *analyze each choice and choose the correct answer*. Chest X-rays are not the study of choice for routine physical exams or for the mass screening of tuberculosis. Furthermore, a chest film should not be taken for every patient that is admitted to the hospital—unless there is suspected cardiopulmonary pathology or an established history of pulmonary disease. Thus, the correct answer is (D)—all of the choices are correct.

Changing Answers That Were Already Correct

Invariably, there will be some questions for which you will choose an answer and then change it. Unfortunately, in doing so you may change some correct answers. Limit such errors by marking each item that you decide to change (place a triangle next to any question to which you changed the answer). Then while reviewing the exam, determine how many questions were changed from right to wrong, wrong to right, and wrong to wrong.

If the majority of answer changes resulted in an increased number of wrong answers, do not change answers during the exam. You are more likely to change answers from right to wrong.

If the majority of answer changes resulted in an increased number of correct questions, then changing answers is actually beneficial.

Finally, if changing answers does not change your score, it means that answers are being changed from wrong to wrong. This indicates that further study is needed in a particular area.

Knowledge Gaps

If a majority of errors relate to a particular topic, you may need to spend additional review time in that area. For example, you might notice that test after test, you tend to miss items that ask you to calculate an answer. This pattern clearly signals its own solution—you must spend more time working with calculations and memorize a few formulas if you want to improve. Perhaps you notice that you often miss items that present a radiograph, and that require you to recognize structures within the film. This signals, again, that you need more visual review. The obvious solution is to adjust your study efforts accordingly, putting more time into and practicing more dynamically with the problematic aspects identified in error analysis.

BEFORE THE EXAM

The following section outlines some practical hints that you can employ in the months, weeks, and days before the exam.

Weeks/Months before the Exam

- Take the practice test in this book to identify areas of strength and weakness.
- Plan a study schedule (be sure to include extra time for areas of weakness).
- Continue to do practice questions (use this book daily).
- Identify other resources that may help with study: group study, study partner, etc.
- Take the online practice test available at kaptest.com\booksonline.

One Week before the Exam

- Do not cram any new material.
- Do not panic if you get practice questions wrong. Instead, use the explanations to clarify details.
- Wake up each day at the same time you will need to awaken on exam day. This will allow you to coordinate your Circadian rhythm.
- Get adequate sleep.
- Do not nap from 8 AM to 5 PM (that would disrupt your Circadian rhythm).
- Visit the testing center to familiarize yourself with the setup.

One Day before the Exam

- Relax. Try to take the day off; if you absolutely must study, then limit yourself to light review.
- Review exam-day basics.
- Get directions to the test center.
- Arrange transportation.
- Arrange for a wake-up call or set the alarm clock.
- Prepare your identification, confirmation number, scheduling permit, personal items, and lunch.
- Get a good night's sleep.

Exam Day

- Have a hearty breakfast. This will provide you with the energy to complete the examination.
- Limit any further review before the test; if you must, do a few practice questions.
- Arrive at the testing center 30 minutes before the scheduled start time of your exam. This will minimize anxiety and ensure that you will not be late.
- Review the decision rules you will employ throughout the test.
- Use relaxation techniques to combat anxiety.
- Utilize a standardized approach when answering each question.

Chapter 3: **Tackling the Computer-Based Test (CBT)**

The American Registry of Radiologic Technologists (ARRT) national certification exam in radiography (the "Registry") is a computer-based test (CBT) that is administered at Pearson VUE test centers across the United States.

THE COMPUTER-BASED TEST

Over the past 10 years, the majority of medical licensure and professional certification exams have adopted computer-based testing. In fact, the ARRT national certification exam has been computerized since 2000. For many student radiographers, the Registry is their first encounter with a computer-based exam. Knowing what to expect will make a significant difference on exam day.

Computer-based testing offers numerous advantages. Exams can be administered at various sites throughout the United States. In addition, examinees are provided with standardized conditions. The physical site, testing interface, and exam content are consistent at all test locations. Furthermore, the rules that govern the behavior and monitoring of examinees are standardized.

Other advantages of a CBT format are increased security and more rapid score reporting. Completed computer-based exams do not need to be shipped back to testing agencies for scoring; instead, examinee data is sent electronically to the testing agency. This reduces the chance of losing grid sheets and exam booklets during shipping. Additionally, examinees receive score reports quicker, usually within two to four weeks of their test date, as compared to the six- to eight-week waiting periods for paper tests.

The future holds even more opportunities that make the CBT attractive. Paper test booklets must be assembled and printed many months before testing dates; therefore, typographic corrections or other changes are difficult to make or must await a new test-creation cycle. With electronically based testing, test developers have quicker and more numerous options for making changes, such as adding images, replacing poor items, or simply correcting typographic mistakes.

Testing software is also changing, as evidenced by the now-routine use of computer adaptive testing (CAT), where item difficulty can be continuously adjusted to the performance of examinees, allowing the testing software to present only as many items as necessary to reach statistical certainty that each individual examinee's knowledge base meets mastery. The advantages of CAT are that items can "live" longer (i.e., remain in use on the test) because they are seen by fewer examinees, and testing sessions can often be shortened, thus freeing space for other examinees to be accommodated within a given period of time. CAT is not currently utilized with the Registry.

As more advanced technology becomes available, test developers look forward to adding even more sophisticated features in the future, including touch-sensitive screens, animated content, and streaming audio and video content. Features such as highlighting text within items, graying out eliminated choices, and continuous availability of item review screens are being developed.

Also note that additional certification exams (e.g., MRI, mammography) are also administered in a CBT format. Thus, the future of medical and allied health licensing exams lies with computer-based testing, and you will benefit from becoming comfortable with it.

SCHEDULING THE EXAM

Most students schedule an exam date that falls within three months of graduation. Once your application is processed by the ARRT, you will be provided with a 90-day window during which time you can take the exam. The testing permit is known as a Candidate Status Report.

If you have not scheduled a date, or if you wish to extend the exam window, simply call the ARRT office at 651-687-0048, ext. 560, for detailed instructions. The request should be honored as long as it is received before your current window expires. The American Registry of Radiologic Technologists will then send you an updated Candidate Status Report.

THE TESTING ENVIRONMENT

Student radiographers take the ARRT national certification exam at Pearson VUE test centers. Students should keep in mind that they will be among a number of other examinees at the center. Several different tests are administered concurrently.

BEFORE YOU LEAVE

Bring the following items with you to the exam:

- Two forms of identification (including one with a current photograph)
- Candidate Status Report issued by the ARRT
- Any medications you may need during the exam
- An extra jacket or sweater

Most test centers will not require a copy of the Candidate Status Report; nonetheless, it is a good idea to have it with you. Except for the identification needed when you check in and an extra jacket/sweater, all other personal items should be left in your car, if possible, because not all center locations have storage lockers for personal items. In any case, you will be allowed to carry only your identification with you into the examination area.

GETTING TO THE TEST CENTER

Arrive at the test center about 30 minutes before your scheduled test appointment to allow time for verification of your credentials and any site-specific introductory information. Visit the test site one week before the examination day—this will reduce test-day anxiety.

WHEN YOU GET THERE

Upon arrival at the center each examinee must present two current forms of identification. (Only one needs to contain a photo. Refer to your Certification Handbook for examples of acceptable forms of identification.) You will then be fingerprinted (for identification purposes) and your picture will be taken. Please make sure that the spelling of your name on these documents is correct. Keep in mind that you will not be given a calculator unless you request one! Remember to request a calculator prior to the start of the exam.

Prior to the examination, each examinee must sign a statement of test center regulations. By signing this statement you agree not to discuss exam content with any other students or examinees. Keep in mind that the testing areas are monitored by video recording.

THE TESTING AREA

Many students comment that the testing areas are either too warm or too cold. Be sure to bring an extra jacket or sweater on exam day.

Food and beverages are not allowed in the testing rooms. The testing rooms are monitored, both electronically and by proctors who walk through the test areas periodically. Once you are brought to the designated test carrel, center staff will start your testing software.

Although center policies are designed to provide all examinees with a comfortable test area equipped with functioning equipment and a reasonably quiet environment, don't expect a sound-proof cubicle. Other types of exams are being given and other examinees may be taking breaks, so you should expect some background noise.

TEST DELIVERY SOFTWARE

The test delivery software is the program that generates the exam for test-takers. The following section presents an overview of the testing interface, answer selection, pilot questions, score reporting, and technical concerns.

TESTING INTERFACE

The testing interface includes all of the items that are visible on the computer screen. Although the ARRT does not provide practice software, the following section describes what you should expect to encounter on exam day.

In terms of questions, many items may include radiographs or drawings. Also, many questions may be lengthy. If the item length exceeds the size of the screen, use the scroll bar to view the entire question. A scroll bar should appear on the right side of the screen. Position the mouse cursor over the scroll, then click and hold to drag the scroll bar.

The following buttons will appear on the screen: Next, Previous, Mark, Review Item, Review Marked Questions, Finished, and Comment.

After you have finished a question, click the **Next** button (in the lower left corner of the screen) to advance to the next question. You may leave items blank and click the **Next** button to advance the test—this is not recommended by Kaplan. Remember, there is no penalty for guessing. You should attempt to answer every question on the exam.

The **Previous** button is located to the right of the Next button. Use it to review questions that have been completed.

The **Mark** button can be used to flag questions to which you would like to return for further review. Kaplan suggests that you limit the use of this feature—you are more likely to complete a question successfully if you answer it on the first pass. It is unlikely that you will have time to review more than a few questions. If you absolutely feel that you should mark an item, select a temporary answer, click on **Mark**, and move on.

When you click the **Review Item** button, a screen with a list of all the items will appear. Click on any item number to link to that question. Ideally, this button should be used only after you have completed the test. Also, any items that have been marked will be obvious.

Simply click **Review Marked Questions** to peruse the items that you had flagged. Once you have completed the section, click **Finished**.

You will have a total of 3.5 hours to complete the 220 questions on the exam. Time remaining is indicated on the screen. Your current question number and total items remaining are also indicated.

Use the timer to pace yourself. You'll have approximately 57 seconds to complete each question. An effective pacing method is to evaluate your performance after each hour of testing—you should complete about 66 questions per hour. Keep track of the remaining time; for example, if you are two hours into the exam and you have not completed 100 questions, you need to answer questions more rapidly.

Another feature of the ARRT examination is the option for test-takers to include comments about individual items during the test itself. Examinees can select the **Comment** button that is located at the bottom of the testing screen; specific comments can then be entered. This feedback will be reviewed by exam authors and members of the ARRT examination committee. Note that the time used to enter comments will be deducted from your remaining test time. Kaplan suggests that comments be made only *after* you complete the exam. In this way, you will not lose valuable testing time.

Students will be provided with a calculator prior to the start of the test, but only on request.

CHOOSING AN ANSWER

Answer selections may be marked in either of two ways:

1. You can position the mouse cursor over the radio button (the circle) for a choice and then click the mouse, which will darken the radio button for that selection.

OR

2. You can use the computer keyboard to press the letter corresponding to your choice and the radio button will darken.

To change your answer using the mouse, just click on the marked radio button (shaded circle), and the mark will disappear. Then you can click another answer choice. To change an answer using the keyboard, simply type the letter of your new selection and the corresponding radio button will be marked.

PILOT QUESTIONS

Pilot or experimental items will be added to the Registry. The data regarding these questions are used by the ARRT to determine whether these questions are useful. Experimental items are not marked in any particular way and will appear as all other questions. About 20 of the 220 total questions will be pilot items. Fortunately, your answers to these questions will not affect your score.

SCORE REPORTING

To pass the Registry, you must achieve a scaled score of 75 on the examination. Basically, you need to correctly answer 66 percent to 67 percent of the questions on the exam. The passing threshold of the exam is known as the "cut score" and is predetermined by the ARRT Board of Trustees.

TECHNICAL CONCERNS

Unfortunately, the ARRT does not provide students with practice materials with which to acclimate themselves to the computer interface. However, the testing interface is intuitive and requires no advanced training. You can answer each question either by clicking the correct choice with the mouse or by typing in the letter of the desired answer choice on the keyboard.

If you experience any technical difficulty with the computer or software during the examination, report it to the test center staff immediately. Often, the exam can be restarted without loss of data. If not, you can reschedule the examination.

FOR ADDITIONAL INFORMATION

Visit the ARRT website, www.arrt.com, for additional information.

Chapter 4: **The Licensure Process**

Most student radiographers complete two years at an accredited radiography program. The two years include both didactic and clinical portions. Upon graduation, students must pass the American Registry of Radiologic Technologists (ARRT) national certification exam (the "Registry"). Subsequently, the radiographer must obtain a state license in order to practice. Currently, *both* registration and licensure are required to practice diagnostic radiography in 35 states.

CERTIFICATION AND REGISTRATION

Certification is the *initial* process that radiographers are required to undertake prior to clinical practice. Essentially, certification is the process whereby radiographers are deemed to have completed the educational requirements, ethical standards, and certification exam administered by the ARRT. A radiographer must keep certification updated with yearly registration.

Certification is a permanent, one-time process. The determinants of eligibility for ARRT certification are ethics, education, and successful completion of the certification examination. Certification is either primary or post-primary. Student radiographers are eligible for *primary certification*.

Primary certification is provided in Radiography, Sonography, Nuclear Medicine Technology, Radiation Therapy, and Magnetic Resonance Imaging. Additionally, post-primary certifications are offered in the following areas: Breast Sonography, Bone Densitometry, Cardiac-Interventional Radiography, Computed Tomography, Mammography, Magnetic Resonance Imaging, Quality Management, Registered Radiologist Assistant, Sonography, Vascular-Interventional Radiography, and Vascular Sonography.

Note that Magnetic Resonance Imaging and Sonography are offered as both primary and post-primary certifications.

The *ethical guidelines* that should be met by prospective clinicians are designed to promote professional conduct and the highest level of ethical behavior while dealing with patients and health care staff. The ARRT requires that you report any prior criminal background—this may not necessarily result in a denial of the application.

In terms of *educational requirements*, prospective radiographers should be graduates of accredited programs. Students should have documented that all didactic and clinical competency requirements have been met. Competence in general patient care and select radiologic procedures should also be documented.

To be certified, the applicant should present a record of educational requirements and ethical standards, and the required fee. Registration also requires that technologists complete a preset number of continuing education (CE) credits each biennium. Thus, the radiographer must demonstrate continued educational effort in the rapidly evolving field of health care. At present, 24 CE credits are required every two years. The majority of the requirement must be *Category A credits*—such educational activities have been evaluated by a Recognized Continuing Education Evaluation Mechanism (RCEEM), such as the American Society of Radiologic Technologists (ASRT).

The current fee for primary certification is $150. ARRT *registration* must be renewed on a yearly basis. Although no exams need to be retaken, the radiographer must meet the eligibility requirements of the ARRT.

Basically, annual registration maintains ARRT certification. Registration with the ARRT allows for the use of the initials R.T. after your name. Some states may not require current registration.

Registration can be conducted online and must be completed prior to the first week of the month prior to the radiographer's birth month. In other words, if a radiographer's birthday is on February 1, he or she should submit the registration materials and fee by January 1. Technologists whose registration is not renewed must apply for reinstatement.

Radiographers can verify registration by checking the ARRT directory on the ARRT website at www.arrt.org, or by phoning the ARRT.

LICENSURE

In addition to ARRT certification and registration, radiologic technologists must be licensed by their respective states to practice. Although laws may differ from state to state, most require a separate state application. Some states may require a score report of your ARRT exam.

Remember, the application for a state license is separate from the ARRT certification application. To determine whether state licensure is necessary to practice, call your state department of health.

SUMMARY

Certification, registration, and licensure can be a confusing process.

1. ARRT certification is a one-time process. It will culminate with the successful completion of the ARRT certification exam.

2. Next, you must acquire a state license. In addition to certification with the ARRT, 35 states require that you possess a state license to practice diagnostic radiography. The application process for a state license is separate from the ARRT certification application. While some states may allow licensure without ARRT certification, it is the exception rather than the rule.

3. Finally, you should keep ARRT certification current by registering with the organization on a yearly basis. This also involves the completion of continuing education (CE) credits every two years. Remember to keep thorough records of all application materials submitted.

PART TWO

Practice Sets

Chapter 5: **Imaging Procedures**

Thorax

1. All of the following structures are considered to be a part of the mediastinum EXCEPT the

   (A) thymus gland.
   (B) lungs.
   (C) trachea.
   (D) esophagus.

2. How many lobes are associated with the right lung?

   (A) 1
   (B) 2
   (C) 3
   (D) 4

3. Which body position would be necessary to obtain an oblique view of the sternum projected into the heart shadow?

   (A) LAO, 45°
   (B) RAO, 45°
   (C) LAO, 15°
   (D) RAO, 15°

4. The diaphragm will move inferiorly with all of the following choices EXCEPT

   (A) inspiration.
   (B) recumbent body position.
   (C) erect body position.
   (D) Fowler's position.

5. Atelectasis is best demonstrated with which of the following radiographs of the chest?

   (A) PA
   (B) Obliques
   (C) Apical lordotic
   (D) Inspiration, expiration

6. The centering point for a PA chest is at which level?

   (A) C7
   (B) T1
   (C) T7
   (D) T12

7. A patient has a barrel chest, there is increased blackening of the lungs, and the lung bases appear to be flattened on the chest radiograph. These are good indications that the patient has which type of condition?

   (A) Emphysema
   (B) Pneumothorax
   (C) Atelectasis
   (D) Asbestosis

8. There are ___ divisions of the pharynx.

   (A) 1
   (B) 2
   (C) 3
   (D) 4

9. Which of the following would be a routine anterior oblique position to visualize an oblique right lung?

   (A) RAO, 15°
   (B) LAO, 15°
   (C) RAO, 45°
   (D) LAO, 45°

10. For demonstration of the apices when the patient is unable to stand for the AP lordotic, how should the central ray be directed?

   (A) 15° cephalad
   (B) 15° caudad
   (C) 45° cephalad
   (D) 45° caudad

Refer to the following radiograph for Questions 11 to 13:

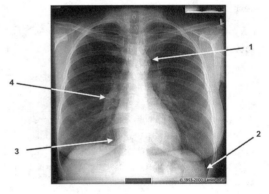

© Copyright DxR Development Group, Inc.

11. Which structure is being identified by Arrow 1?

   (A) Aortic arch
   (B) Hilum
   (C) Left ventricle
   (D) Left subclavian artery

12. Which arrow identifies a cardiophrenic angle?

   (A) 1
   (B) 2
   (C) 3
   (D) 4

13. All of the following structures are located within the dense area indicated by Arrow 4 EXCEPT the

   (A) bronchi.
   (B) pulmonary vessels.
   (C) lymph vessels.
   (D) pleura.

14. Which numbered pair of ribs is associated with costotransverse joints?

   (A) 1–7
   (B) 1–10
   (C) 8–12
   (D) 11 and 12

15. Which of the following would be the anterior oblique position and patient instruction utilized for demonstration of the right axillary ribs above the diaphragm?

   (A) RAO, inspiration
   (B) LAO, inspiration
   (C) RAO, expiration
   (D) LAO, inspiration

16. The leaf-shaped flap of cartilage that covers the laryngeal opening is the

   (A) glottis.
   (B) epiglottis.
   (C) cricoid cartilage.
   (D) thyroid cartilage.

GO ON TO THE NEXT PAGE

Refer to the following image for Questions 17 to 20:

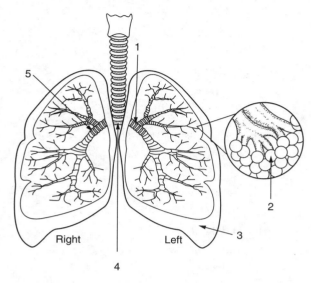

Right   Left

17. Arrow 2 represents which of the following structures?

(A) Alveoli

(B) Bronchioles

(C) Bronchi

(D) Pleura

18. If a patient swallows a foreign object the size of a coin, it is most likely to become lodged in the portion of the respiratory system indicated by which numbered arrow?

(A) 1

(B) 2

(C) 4

(D) 5

19. Which of the following conditions exists if there is an abnormal accumulation of fluid in the structure being identified by Arrow 3?

(A) Atelectasis

(B) Pneumothorax

(C) Pleural effusion

(D) Bronchitis

20. What is the level of the structure identified by Arrow 4?

(A) C7

(B) T1

(C) T5

(D) T10

Abdomen and GI Studies

1. The longest segment of the small intestine is the

(A) cecum.

(B) duodenum.

(C) ileum.

(D) jejunum.

2. Which is the portion of the alimentary canal where digestion and the absorption of food occur?

(A) Esophagus

(B) Stomach

(C) Large intestine

(D) Small intestine

3. When performing a double-contrast barium enema, which position will BEST demonstrate the lateral aspect of the descending colon?

(A) Supine

(B) Prone

(C) Right lateral decubitus

(D) Left lateral decubitus

4. What is the term that describes the telescoping of bowel into a distal segment?

(A) Intussusception

(B) Volvulus

(C) Ileus

(D) Varices

GO ON TO THE NEXT PAGE

KAPLAN

5. When performing a double-contrast gastrointestinal examination of the stomach, for demonstration of an air-filled fundus, it is BEST to have the patient in which of the following positions?

   1. Supine
   2. Posterior oblique
   3. Anterior oblique

   (A) 1 only
   (B) 3 only
   (C) 1 and 2 only
   (D) 1 and 3 only

Refer to the following radiograph for Questions 6 and 7:

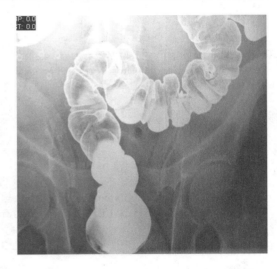

6. To obtain an image as in the radiograph above, with the patient prone, it is BEST to direct the central ray in which degree and direction?

   (A) 15° cephalad
   (B) 15° caudad
   (C) 30° cephalad
   (D) 30° caudad

7. The anatomy imaged above is a portion of which larger structure?

   (A) Esophagus
   (B) Stomach
   (C) Small intestine
   (D) Large intestine

8. The patient does not orally ingest the contrast medium for which of the following studies of the small intestine?

   1. Small bowel series
   2. Enteroclysis procedure
   3. Intubation method

   (A) 1 and 2 only
   (B) 1 and 3 only
   (C) 2 and 3 only
   (D) 1, 2, and 3

9. Which of the following body positions will demonstrate anterior and posterior aspects of the stomach on the same image?

   (A) AP
   (B) RAO
   (C) RPO
   (D) Lateral

GO ON TO THE NEXT PAGE

Refer to the following image for Questions 10 to 13:

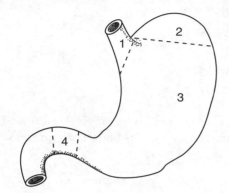

10. Which numbered structure has the majority of the lesser and greater curvatures as its borders?

    (A) 1
    (B) 2
    (C) 3
    (D) 4

11. Which numbered structure represents the portion of the stomach where the cardiac sphincter is located?

    (A) 1
    (B) 2
    (C) 3
    (D) 4

12. During an upper GI examination, to demonstrate numbered structure 4 most actively emptying, it is best to have the patient in which body position?

    (A) Supine
    (B) RAO
    (C) LAO
    (D) LPO

13. The radiographic sign of Schatzki's ring is associated with which of the following?

    (A) Sliding hiatal hernia
    (B) Acute gastritis
    (C) Diverticula
    (D) Bezoars

14. The cecum is located in which quadrant of the abdomen?

    (A) Right upper quadrant
    (B) Right lower quadrant
    (C) Left upper quadrant
    (D) Left lower quadrant

15. During a small bowel series, spot films are usually obtained when the contrast reaches which region?

    (A) Pyloric sphincter
    (B) Ileocecal valve
    (C) Jejunum
    (D) Duodenum

16. Which section of the alimentary canal contains pouches termed haustrum?

    (A) Esophagus
    (B) Stomach
    (C) Small intestine
    (D) Large intestine

17. During a double-contrast barium enema, which portions of the large intestine are MOST likely to fill with air when the patient is in the supine position?

    1. Transverse colon
    2. Ascending colon
    3. Sigmoid colon

    (A) 1 and 2 only
    (B) 1 and 3 only
    (C) 2 and 3 only
    (D) 1, 2, and 3

GO ON TO THE NEXT PAGE

18. Which anterior oblique position BEST demonstrates the left colic flexure without superimposition?

    (A) RAO, 45°

    (B) LAO, 45°

    (C) RAO, 60°

    (D) LAO, 60°

Refer to the following radiograph for Questions 19 and 20:

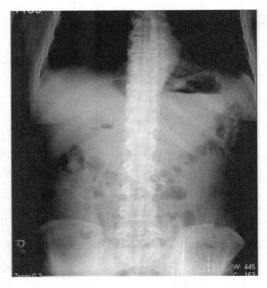

19. What is the patient position utilized to obtain this image?

    (A) Supine

    (B) Prone

    (C) Erect

    (D) Lateral decubitus

20. If the patient were unable to achieve the position demonstrated above, what would be the alternative solution for visualization of structures?

    (A) Supine

    (B) Prone

    (C) Trendelenburg

    (D) Lateral decubitus

21. Which is the correct level of centering for an AP supine abdomen?

    (A) T9–10

    (B) L2–3

    (C) L4–5

    (D) S1–2

22. Which of the following images do NOT need to be obtained for a single-contrast barium enema?

    (A) Lateral rectum

    (B) Left and right decubitus

    (C) RPO

    (D) LPO

23. During a single-contrast gastrointestinal series, which patient position is sometimes used to better demonstrate a sliding hiatal hernia?

    (A) Trendelenburg

    (B) Fowler's

    (C) Sims'

    (D) Upright

24. In the sequence of images taken for a double-contrast barium enema, visualization of the outline of the mucosal pattern of the large intestine occurs with which image?

    (A) RAO

    (B) LAO

    (C) Lateral

    (D) PA, post-evacuation

25. Which radiographic examinations could include images of the esophagus?

    1. Barium swallow
    2. Upper GI
    3. Lower GI

    (A) 1 only

    (B) 1 and 2 only

    (C) 2 and 3 only

    (D) 1, 2, and 3

GO ON TO THE NEXT PAGE ▷

26. Of the following, which is the most proximal structure of the alimentary canal?

    (A) Esophagus

    (B) Stomach

    (C) Small intestine

    (D) Large intestine

Refer to the following radiograph for Questions 27 and 28:

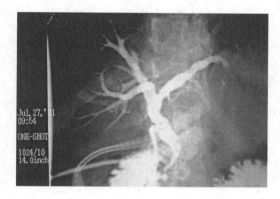

27. According to evidence demonstrated in the radiograph above, which radiographic procedure is being performed?

    (A) ERCP

    (B) Oral cholecystogram

    (C) Enteroclysis procedure

    (D) Retrograde pyelogram

28. What does the procedure being demonstrated best evaluate?

    (A) Biliary and pancreatic ducts

    (B) Kidneys and ureters

    (C) Duodenum

    (D) Liver function

29. During an esophagram, in the RAO position, where should the esophagus appear on the image?

    (A) Between the heart and the vertebral column

    (B) Superimposed on the scapula

    (C) Superimposed on the vertebral column

    (D) Superimposed on the heart shadow

30. During an upper gastrointestinal examination of a sthenic patient, which is the proper degree of obliquity to BEST visualize the stomach?

    (A) 15°

    (B) 25°

    (C) 45°

    (D) 70°

31. What is the wavelike contraction of the muscles in the alimentary canal termed?

    (A) Deglutition

    (B) Peristalsis

    (C) Evacuation

    (D) Mastication

Urologic Studies

1. In which position is the patient placed for retrograde urography?

    (A) Modified lithotomy

    (B) Trendelenburg

    (C) Fowler's

    (D) Sims'

2. Which of the following will BEST demonstrate enlargement of the prostate when performing an IVP?

    (A) AP, ureteric compression

    (B) PA

    (C) AP upright, post-void

    (D) LPO and RPO

GO ON TO THE NEXT PAGE ⇒

KAPLAN

3. Which of the following pathologies will affect normal form of the structure of the kidneys, but NOT its function?

    (A) Hydronephrosis

    (B) Polycystic kidney disease

    (C) Nephrosclerosis

    (D) Horseshoe kidneys

4. What is the most common position in which the male patient is placed for voiding cystoure-thrography?

    (A) 30°, RPO

    (B) 30°, LPO

    (C) 45°, RPO

    (D) 45°, LPO

5. During intravenous urography, to capture the contrast within the nephron phase, the image should be taken how many minutes after the injection of contrast media?

    (A) 1

    (B) 5

    (C) 15

    (D) 30

6. What are the most common sites where kidney stones become lodged?

    1. Pelvic brim
    2. Ureteropelvic junction
    3. Ureterovesical junction

    (A) 1 only

    (B) 1 and 2 only

    (C) 2 and 3 only

    (D) 1, 2, and 3

7. What is the correct degree of patient obliquity for obliques of the bladder?

    (A) 5°

    (B) 15°

    (C) 30°

    (D) 60°

8. When is a ureteric compression band contraindi-cated?

    1. Abdominal mass
    2. Abdominal surgery
    3. Ureteric stones

    (A) 1 only

    (B) 1 and 3 only

    (C) 2 and 3 only

    (D) 1, 2, and 3

9. What is the correct oblique for best demonstration of the right kidney during an IVP?

    (A) RPO, 45°

    (B) LPO, 45°

    (C) RPO, 30°

    (D) LPO, 30°

10. What is the direction of the central ray for an AP of the urinary bladder?

    (A) 15° cephalad

    (B) 15° caudad

    (C) 30° cephalad

    (D) 30° caudad

11. Which of the following measures the functional aspect of the urinary system?

    1. Intravenous urography
    2. Retrograde urography
    3. Retrograde cystography

    (A) 1 only

    (B) 3 only

    (C) 1 and 2 only

    (D) 2 and 3 only

GO ON TO THE NEXT PAGE ⟩

12. Which of the following is a functional study of the bladder and urethra?

    (A) Intravenous urography
    (B) Retrograde urography
    (C) Retrograde cystogram
    (D) Voiding cystourethrogram

Refer to the following image for Questions 13 to 15:

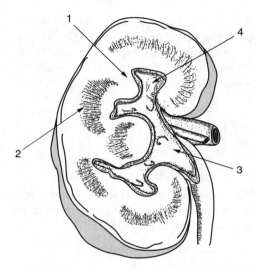

13. What number points to the collection portion that is just proximal to the ureter and lies within the hilum of the kidney?

    (A) 1
    (B) 2
    (C) 3
    (D) 4

14. Arrow 4 is pointing to the

    (A) major calyx.
    (B) renal cortex.
    (C) renal pyramid.
    (D) renal pelvis.

15. Which arrow identifies the portion of the kidney that is composed of collecting tubules?

    (A) 1
    (B) 2
    (C) 3
    (D) 4

Spine and Pelvis

1. Which of the following is NOT one of the bones that fuses to form the acetabulum?

    (A) Sacrum
    (B) Ilium
    (C) Ischium
    (D) Pubis

2. What is the relationship between structures when obtaining a cross-table lateral hip?

    (A) Central ray parallel to femoral neck and image receptor
    (B) Central ray perpendicular to femoral neck and image receptor
    (C) Central ray perpendicular with long axis of femur and parallel with image receptor
    (D) Central ray parallel with long axis of femur and perpendicular to image receptor

GO ON TO THE NEXT PAGE

Refer to the following radiograph for Questions 3 and 4:

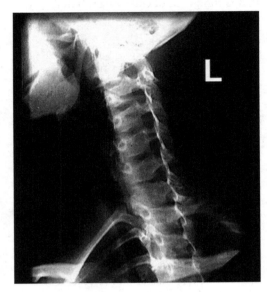

© Copyright DxR Development Group, Inc.

3. If the radiograph above is a PA oblique projection, which of the following is TRUE of how the image was obtained?

    (A) 15° cephalad central ray, RAO body position

    (B) 15° caudad central ray, RAO body position

    (C) 15° cephalad central ray, LAO body position

    (D) 15° caudad central ray, LAO body position

4. To obtain the image above, the patient was obliqued how many degrees?

    (A) 15°

    (B) 30°

    (C) 45°

    (D) 60°

5. Which projection of the lumbar spine follows the lumbar curve for BEST demonstration of the intervertebral disk space?

    (A) AP

    (B) PA

    (C) Lateral

    (D) AP obliques

6. For the BEST demonstration of the left lumbar zygapophyseal joints with a PA oblique projection, it is necessary to have the patient in which body position?

    (A) RAO, 45°

    (B) LAO, 45°

    (C) RAO, 70°

    (D) LAO, 70°

7. A patient is injured by diving into a shallow pool. The open-mouth image of the cervical spine reveals a spreading of the lateral masses of C1 relative to the dens. It is MOST likely that the patient has which type of fracture?

    (A) Clay shoveler's

    (B) Jefferson

    (C) Hangman's

    (D) Teardrop

8. The radiographic appearance of a collar around the "Scotty dog" on an oblique lumbar spine image is a sign of which defect?

    (A) Anklyosing spondylitis

    (B) Spondylolysis

    (C) Osteogenesis imperfecta

    (D) Spina bifida

9. To visualize the left acetabulum utilizing the Judet method, what is the degree of obliquity of the patient?

    (A) 15°

    (B) 30°

    (C) 45°

    (D) 60°

GO ON TO THE NEXT PAGE

10. Which of the following portions of the spinal column have a lordotic curvature?

 1. Cervical spine
 2. Thoracic spine
 3. Lumbar spine

 (A) 1 only
 (B) 2 only
 (C) 2 and 3 only
 (D) 1 and 3 only

11. For best visualization of the right sacroiliac joint with an AP oblique projection, the patient should be placed in which body position?

 (A) RPO, 25 to 30°
 (B) LPO, 25 to 30°
 (C) RPO, 45°
 (D) LPO, 45°

wrong in book

12. Patient condition permitting, when taking an AP pelvis radiograph it is necessary to rotate the lower extremities into which position to place the femoral necks parallel with the plane of the image receptor?

 (A) 5 to 10° internally
 (B) 5 to 10° externally
 (C) 15 to 20° internally
 (D) 15 to 20° externally

13. The ear of the "Scotty dog" on an oblique lumbar spine radiograph corresponds to which portion of the lumbar vertebra anatomy?

 (A) Superior articular facet
 (B) Lamina
 (C) Pars interarticularis
 (D) Pedicle

wrong in book

Refer to the following image for Questions 14 and 15:

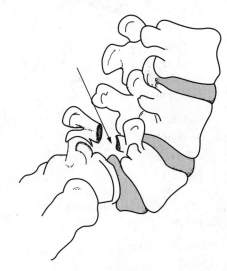

14. In the image above, the arrow is identifying which portion of bone associated with the lumbar spine?

 (A) Superior articular facet
 (B) Inferior articular facet
 (C) Spinous process
 (D) Pars interarticularis

15. What condition associated with the lumbar spine is represented in the above image?

 (A) Ankylosing spondylitis
 (B) Spondylolysis
 (C) Spondylolisthesis
 (D) Spina bifida

GO ON TO THE NEXT PAGE →

KAPLAN)

16. If the patient has a suspected hip fracture, which of the following could be utilized for a lateral view of the femoral neck?

    1. Unilateral frog-leg
    2. Cross-table lateral
    3. Axiolateral inferosuperior (Clements-Nakayama)

    (A) 1 only
    (B) 1 and 3 only
    (C) 2 and 3 only
    (D) 1, 2, and 3

17. Which of the following BEST demonstrates congenital hip dislocation?

    (A) Bilateral frog-leg
    (B) AP pelvis
    (C) AP, inlet/outlet
    (D) Posterior oblique, Judet

18. When obtaining a lateral image of L5-S1, if there is lumbar sag present, how should the central ray be directed to open the joint space?

    (A) 5° caudad
    (B) 5° cephalad
    (C) 15° caudad
    (D) 15° cephalad

19. There are how many segments of the adult sacrum?

    (A) 2
    (B) 3
    (C) 4
    (D) 5

20. To include the sacrum and coccyx on one lateral image, where should the central ray be directed?

    (A) To the midcoronal plane
    (B) To the ASIS
    (C) 2 inches posterior to the ASIS
    (D) 3–4 inches posterior to the ASIS

Refer to the following image for Questions 21 to 24:

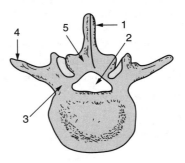

21. Which portion of this lumbar vertebra is represented by Arrow 5?

    (A) Spinous process
    (B) Lamina
    (C) Pedicle
    (D) Transverse process

22. In the articulated vertebral column, the inferior and superior surfaces of the structure identified by Arrow 3 form which of the following?

    (A) Intervertebral foramina
    (B) Costotransverse joints
    (C) Vertebral foramina
    (D) Zygapophyseal joints

GO ON TO THE NEXT PAGE

23. Which numbered structure represents the transverse process?

    (A) 1

    (B) 3

    (C) 4

    (D) 5

24. Which numbered structure represents the spinous process?

    (A) 1

    (B) 3

    (C) 4

    (D) 5

25. What is the correct angle and direction of the central ray for an AP projection of the coccyx?

    (A) 10° cephalad

    (B) 10° caudad

    (C) 15° cephalad

    (D) 15° caudad

26. Which is the best position to demonstrate the intervertebral foramina of the thoracic spine?

    (A) AP

    (B) Lateral

    (C) 45° obliques

    (D) 60° obliques

27. To position the PA dens (Judd), which positioning line is placed perpendicular to the plane of the image receptor?

    (A) OML

    (B) IOML

    (C) AML

    (D) MML

28. To demonstrate the L5–S1 interspace with an AP projection, how is the central ray angled?

    (A) 15° cephalad

    (B) 15° caudad

    (C) 30° cephalad

    (D) 30° caudad

29. The lateral aspect of the greater trochanter of the femur is in line with which structure?

    (A) Pubic symphysis

    (B) Iliac crest

    (C) Sacrum

    (D) ASIS

Refer to the following radiograph for Questions 30 to 33:

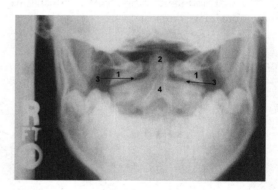

30. Which portion of bone does Number 1 identify?

    (A) Pedicles

    (B) Laminae

    (C) Lateral masses

    (D) Spinous process

31. Which portion of bone does Number 4 identify?

    (A) Pedicles

    (B) Laminae

    (C) Lateral masses

    (D) Spinous process

GO ON TO THE NEXT PAGE

KAPLAN

32. What anatomy is being identified by Arrow 3?

    (A) Zygapophyseal joints
    (B) Intervertebral foramina
    (C) Cervical foramina
    (D) Atlantooccipital joints

33. What is the correct relationship of structures to obtain the position necessary for producing this image of the cervical spine?

    (A) Lower edge of incisors and EAM are perpendicular to the image receptor.
    (B) Lower edge of incisors and mastoid tip are perpendicular to image receptor.
    (C) AML and EAM are perpendicular to the image receptor.
    (D) AML and mastoid tip are perpendicular to the image receptor.

Cranium

1. How many bones are located within the skull?

    (A) 8
    (B) 14
    (C) 22
    (D) 25

2. The crista galli is a conical projection that arises from which bone?

    (A) Ethmoid
    (B) Sphenoid
    (C) Temporal
    (D) Occipital

3. Which of the following projections best demonstrates the maxillary sinuses?

    (A) Parietoacanthial (Waters)
    (B) PA axial (Caldwell)
    (C) SMV (full basal)
    (D) Lateral

Refer to the following image for Questions 4 to 7:

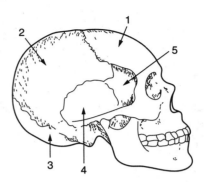

4. The PA projection of the skull best demonstrates the bone identified by which number?

    (A) 1
    (B) 2
    (C) 3
    (D) 4

5. The sella turcica is located as part of the bone identified by which number?

    (A) 2
    (B) 3
    (C) 4
    (D) 5

6. The organs of hearing are located within which numbered structure?

    (A) 1
    (B) 2
    (C) 3
    (D) 4

7. The foramen magnum is located within which numbered structure?

    (A) 2
    (B) 3
    (C) 4
    (D) 5

GO ON TO THE NEXT PAGE

8. Which is true of the lateral (Law) for demonstration of TMJs when the skull is placed in a true lateral position?

    (A) The face is rotated 15° toward the image receptor, central ray 15° caudad.

    (B) The face is rotated 15° toward the image receptor, central ray 15° cephalad.

    (C) The face is rotated 15° away from the image receptor, central ray 15° caudad.

    (D) The face is rotated 15° away from the image receptor, central ray 15° cephalad.

9. For the PA axial (Caldwell), for facial bones, how is the central ray directed?

    (A) 15° cephalad, exit nasion

    (B) 15° caudad, exit nasion

    (C) 15° cephalad, exit acanthion

    (D) 15° caudad, exit acanthion

10. Which of the following projections can be utilized to demonstrate the zygomatic arches?

    1. Parietoacanthial (Waters)
    2. Submentovertical
    3. AP axial (Towne)

    (A) 1 only

    (B) 1 and 3 only

    (C) 2 and 3 only

    (D) 1, 2, and 3

11. Which projection will demonstrate the cranial base?

    (A) Parietoacanthial (Waters)

    (B) PA axial (Caldwell)

    (C) AP axial (Towne)

    (D) Submentovertical

Refer to the following image for Questions 12 and 13:

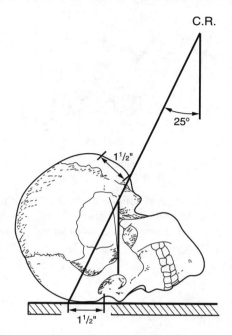

12. Utilizing the projection demonstrated by the figure above, which bone is visualized BEST?

    (A) Frontal

    (B) Maxilla

    (C) Occipital

    (D) Parietal

13. When the projection demonstrated above cannot be obtained as a PA axial, the alternative for the same demonstration in the AP axial projection will be how many degrees caudad when the orbitomeatal line is perpendicular to the plane of the image receptor?

    (A) 25°

    (B) 30°

    (C) 37°

    (D) 15°

GO ON TO THE NEXT PAGE ⟩

Refer to the following image for Questions 14 to 16:

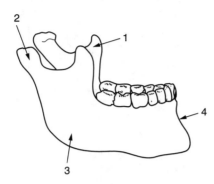

14. For an axiolateral oblique to demonstrate the anatomy identified by Arrow 4, the head must be rotated how many degrees from lateral toward the image receptor?

    (A) 0°
    (B) 15°
    (C) 30°
    (D) 45°

15. What is the process identified by Arrow 1?

    (A) Coronoid
    (B) Coracoid
    (C) Condyloid
    (D) Styloid

16. The structure identified by Arrow 2 meets with which bone to form its articulation?

    (A) Frontal
    (B) Parietal
    (C) Temporal
    (D) Sphenoid

17. What is the projection that will demonstrate the petrous ridges within the lower third of the orbits when the OML is perpendicular to the image receptor?

    (A) PA axial, 15° caudad
    (B) PA axial, 15° cephalad
    (C) PA axial, 25° caudad
    (D) PA axial, 25° cephalad

18. Which bone is NOT considered to be a paired bone of the face?

    (A) Maxilla
    (B) Palatine
    (C) Lacrimal
    (D) Vomer

19. If a patient has a tripod fracture, which bone comes free from its articulations?

    (A) Maxillary
    (B) Mandible
    (C) Palatine
    (D) Zygoma

20. For the best demonstration of a blowout fracture to the orbits, the OML should be placed how many degrees from the plane of the image receptor?

    (A) 15°
    (B) 30°
    (C) 37°
    (D) 45°

21. For the best demonstration of the proximal rami and condyloid process of the mandible with a PA projection, the central ray should be angled which way?

    (A) 25° cephalad
    (B) 25° caudad
    (C) 15° cephalad
    (D) 15° caudad

22. Which sinuses are demonstrated through the open-mouth parietoacanthial (Waters)?

    (A) Frontal
    (B) Sphenoid
    (C) Ethmoid
    (D) Maxillary

GO ON TO THE NEXT PAGE

23. There is evidence of tilt on a lateral skull radiograph when which of the following is NOT placed truly perpendicular to the plane of the image receptor?

    (A) Interpupillary line
    (B) Infraorbitomeatal line
    (C) Orbitomeatal line
    (D) Midsagittal plane

24. The sphenoid sinuses will be demonstrated without superimposition on which of the following radiographs of the paranasal sinuses?

    1. Lateral
    2. Submentovertical
    3. PA Axial (Caldwell)

    (A) 1 only
    (B) 1 and 2 only
    (C) 2 and 3 only
    (D) 3 only

Extremities

Refer to the following image for Questions 1 to 3:

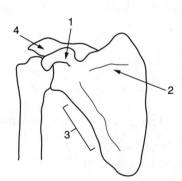

1. Arrow 1 identifies which process of the scapula?

    (A) Acromion
    (B) Coracoid
    (C) Coronoid
    (D) Condyloid

2. Which fossa is identified by Arrow 2?

    (A) Subscapular
    (B) Subclavicular
    (C) Supraspinous
    (D) Infraspinous

3. Which border is identified by Number 3?

    (A) Superior
    (B) Inferior
    (C) Medial
    (D) Lateral

4. For the AP oblique foot, medial rotation, the plantar surface forms an angle of how many degrees to the plane of the image receptor?

    (A) 15°
    (B) 30°
    (C) 45°
    (D) 50°

5. The proper movement of the arm for positioning of an AP forearm is

    (A) eversion.
    (B) inversion.
    (C) supination.
    (D) pronation.

6. Which projection of the elbow demonstrates the olecranon process in profile?

    (A) AP
    (B) AP oblique, internal rotation
    (C) AP oblique, external rotation
    (D) Lateral

GO ON TO THE NEXT PAGE

7. What is the proper central ray angulation for a plantodorsal projection of the calcaneus?

   (A) 15°
   (B) 30°
   (C) 40°
   (D) 60°

8. How many interphalangeal joints are there in the first digit?

   (A) 1
   (B) 2
   (C) 3
   (D) 4

9. Which of the following projections BEST demonstrates the longitudinal arch of the foot?

   (A) AP, non-weight-bearing
   (B) AP oblique, medial rotation
   (C) Lateral, non-weight-bearing
   (D) AP and lateral, weight-bearing

10. To visualize the interphalangeal joints of the toes as open with an AP projection, the central ray is angled how many degrees posteriorly?

    (A) 0°
    (B) 10°
    (C) 15°
    (D) 30°

Refer to the following radiograph for Questions 11 to 14:

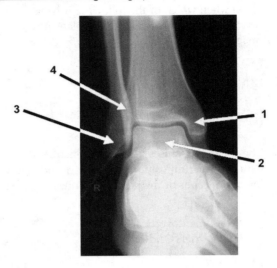

11. What is the rotation of the lower extremity to produce the image as seen above?

    (A) 15° internal
    (B) 15° external
    (C) 45° internal
    (D) 45° external

12. Which arrow identifies the talus?

    (A) 1
    (B) 2
    (C) 3
    (D) 4

13. Which articulation is identified by Arrow 4?

    (A) Proximal tibiofibular
    (B) Distal tibiofibular
    (C) Tibiotalar
    (D) Talofibular

GO ON TO THE NEXT PAGE ▷

14. Which structure is identified by Arrow 1?

    (A) Medial malleolus

    (B) Lateral malleolus

    (C) Medial condyle

    (D) Lateral condyle

15. Which of the following carpal bones is the most lateral?

    (A) Scaphoid

    (B) Capitate

    (C) Triquetrum

    (D) Pisiform

16. What is the centering point for a PA of the hand?

    (A) 2nd proximal interphalangeal joint

    (B) 3rd proximal interphalangeal joint

    (C) 2nd metacarpophalangeal joint

    (D) 3rd metacarpophalangeal joint

17. What is the BEST projection of the knee for demonstration of Osgood-Schlatter's disease?

    (A) AP oblique, lateral rotation

    (B) AP oblique, medial rotation

    (C) Tangential (Settegast)

    (D) Lateral

18. Which of the following projections of the hand places the thumb in an oblique position?

    (A) PA

    (B) PA oblique, external rotation

    (C) Lateral in extension

    (D) Lateral in flexion

19. When an asthenic patient is standing erect for an AP axial projection of the clavicle, the proper central ray angulation is which of the following?

    (A) 10° caudad

    (B) 10° cephalad

    (C) 30° caudad

    (D) 30° cephalad

Refer to the following image for Questions 20 to 22:

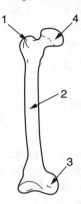

20. Which structure is identified by Arrow 1?

    (A) Medial condyle

    (B) Lateral condyle

    (C) Greater trochanter

    (D) Lesser trochanter

21. The femoral head is identified by which arrow?

    (A) 1

    (B) 2

    (C) 3

    (D) 4

22. The structure identified by Arrow 2 is which portion of bone in an adolescent?

    (A) Epiphysis

    (B) Epiphyseal plate

    (C) Diaphysis

    (D) Articular end

23. Which of the following projections will demonstrate a lateral view of the proximal humerus if the patient is unable to rotate or abduct his or her upper extremity?

    (A) Inferosuperior axial

    (B) Tangential

    (C) Posterior oblique (Grashey)

    (D) Transthoracic lateral

GO ON TO THE NEXT PAGE

KAPLAN

24. For proper visualization of the _____ articulation, it is necessary to acquire two images—one with the patient holding 8- to 10-pound weights, one without the patient holding any weight.

    (A) sternoclavicular
    (B) acromioclavicular
    (C) glenohumeral
    (D) humeroulnar

25. For demonstration of the scaphoid (Stecher), with the wrist parallel to the image receptor, how should the central ray be angled?

    (A) 20° toward elbow
    (B) 20° toward fingers
    (C) 30° toward elbow
    (D) 30° toward fingers

26. For the scapular Y projection, the midcoronal plane forms an angle of how many degrees to the plane of the image receptor?

    (A) 10–20°
    (B) 25–30°
    (C) 45–60°
    (D) 65–75°

27. The proper centering point for an AP shoulder is which of the following?

    (A) 1 inch superior to the coracoid process
    (B) 2 inches superior to the coracoid process
    (C) 1 inch inferior to the coracoid process
    (D) 3 inches inferior to the coracoid process

28. To demonstrate the greater tubercle in profile on a projection of the humerus, the hand should be

    (A) pronated.
    (B) supinated.
    (C) neutral.
    (D) lateral.

29. The sustentaculum tali is a portion of which of the following tarsal bones?

    (A) Calcaneus
    (B) Cuboid
    (C) Navicular
    (D) Talus

30. Which projection of the hand demonstrates an anterior or posterior displacement of a fracture?

    (A) PA
    (B) PA, external rotation
    (C) PA, internal rotation
    (D) Lateral

GO ON TO THE NEXT PAGE

Refer to the following radiograph for Questions 31 to 33:

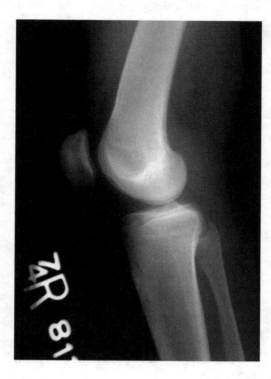

31.

What is the routine degree of flexion utilized for the projection demonstrated above?

(A) 5°

(B) 20–30°

(C) 45°

(D) 55–65°

32. If properly positioned, which of the following articulations will be demonstrated in this view?

1. Patellofemoral
2. Femorotibial
3. Proximal tibiofibular

(A) 1 only

(B) 1 and 2 only

(C) 2 and 3 only

(D) 1, 2, and 3

33. For the routine projection seen in the radiograph above, the central ray should be directed

(A) 5 to 7° cephalad

(B) 5 to 7° caudad

(C) 15° cephalad

(D) 15° caudad

34. The sesamoid bones of the foot are demonstrated without superimposition on which projection?

(A) AP

(B) Medial oblique

(C) Lateral oblique

(D) Tangential

35. What is the central ray angle for a mediolateral projection of the calcaneus?

(A) 0°

(B) 15°

(C) 30°

(D) 40°

36. For which of the following studies is a PA projection of the left hand taken to evaluate ossification centers?

(A) Bone age

(B) Bone survey

(C) Long-bone measurement

(D) Soft-tissue study

37. Which of the following projections place the epicondyles of the distal humerus parallel to the plane of the image receptor?

1. AP humerus
2. lateral elbow
3. AP shoulder, external rotation

(A) 2 only

(B) 3 only

(C) 1 and 3 only

(D) 1, 2, and 3

GO ON TO THE NEXT PAGE

38. How many articulations are there between the tibia and fibula?

    (A) 1
    (B) 2
    (C) 3
    (D) 4

39. To demonstrate the patella with the patient prone and the leg flexed 90°, how many degrees cephalad should the central ray be directed?

    (A) 5°
    (B) 15–20°
    (C) 30–40°
    (D) 55°

40. For an AP projection of the thumb, the hand is

    (A) internally rotated.
    (B) externally rotated.
    (C) hyperextended.
    (D) acutely flexed.

Refer to the following image for Questions 41 to 43:

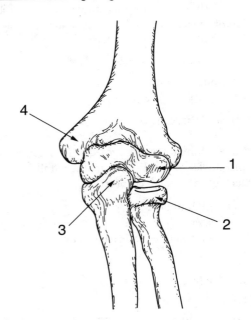

41. Arrow 3 above identifies a structure that is seen in profile with which projection of the elbow?

    (A) AP
    (B) AP oblique, medial rotation
    (C) AP oblique, lateral rotation
    (D) Lateral

42. Which arrow identifies the medial epicondyle?

    (A) 1
    (B) 2
    (C) 3
    (D) 4

43. Which structure is identified by Arrow 2?

    (A) Styloid process of ulna
    (B) Styloid process of radius
    (C) Head of ulna
    (D) Head of radius

44. For the dorsoplantar projection of the foot, the central ray is angled posteriorly how many degrees?

    (A) 5°
    (B) 10°
    (C) 15°
    (D) 20°

45. The interspace between the medial and intermediate cuneiforms are visualized free of superimposition in which projection?

    (A) AP
    (B) AP oblique, medial rotation
    (C) AP oblique, lateral rotation
    (D) Lateral

GO ON TO THE NEXT PAGE

46. Which projection of the ankle helps to demonstrate the rupture of a ligament?

    (A) AP

    (B) AP, stress views

    (C) AP, weight-bearing

    (D) Lateral

47. There is an open joint space demonstrated between the humeral head and the glenoid cavity in which projection?

    (A) AP, internal rotation

    (B) AP, external rotation

    (C) AP oblique projection (Grashey)

    (D) Scapular Y

48. What is the proper movement of the foot for a lateral projection of the ankle?

    (A) Dorsiflexion

    (B) Plantarflexion

    (C) Eversion

    (D) Inversion

49. A trimalleolar fracture involves which of the following bones?

    (A) Femur

    (B) Humerus

    (C) Tibia, fibula

    (D) Radius, ulna

Refer to the following radiograph for Questions 50 to 52:

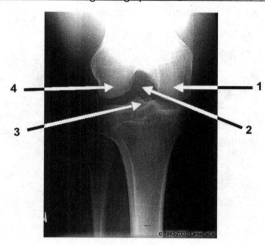

© Copyright DxR Development Group, Inc.

50. The radiograph above is which projection?

    (A) AP knee

    (B) AP, weight-bearing

    (C) AP oblique, medial rotation

    (D) PA axial, intercondylar fossa

51. Which arrow indentifies intercondylar eminences?

    (A) 1

    (B) 2

    (C) 3

    (D) 4

52. Which structure is identified by Arrow 4?

    (A) Medial epicondyle

    (B) Lateral epicondyle

    (C) Medial condyle

    (D) Lateral condyle

GO ON TO THE NEXT PAGE

KAPLAN

53. How should the lower extremity be rotated for an AP projection of the proximal femur?

    (A) 15° medially
    (B) 15° laterally
    (C) 45° medially
    (D) 45° laterally

54. The femoral condyles are placed parallel with the image receptor for which projection?

    (A) AP lower leg
    (B) AP oblique, medial rotation
    (C) Lateral ankle
    (D) Lateral lower leg

55. What is the flexion of the affected knee for a lateral patella?

    (A) 5–10°
    (B) 20–30°
    (C) 45°
    (D) 55–65°

56. Which projection of the elbow requires two radiographs to be taken—one with the distal humerus parallel to the image receptor, one with the proximal forearm parallel?

    (A) AP
    (B) AP, partial flexion
    (C) AP, obliques
    (D) lateral

57. The fibula will be superimposed on the posterior half of the tibia on which projection?

    (A) AP
    (B) AP oblique, medial rotation
    (C) AP oblique, lateral rotation
    (D) Mediolateral

58. To BEST demonstrate the body on a lateral projection of the scapula, the patient's affected arm is in which of the following positions?

    (A) Neutral
    (B) Across the front of the chest, grasping the opposite shoulder
    (C) Flexed behind the back, partially abducted
    (D) At the side, externally rotated

59. For the carpal canal projection, when the patient hyperextends the wrist, the central ray is directed how many degrees to the long axis of the hand?

    (A) 5°
    (B) 10–15°
    (C) 25–30°
    (D) 45°

60. What classification of joint is the first carpometacarpal joint?

    (A) Ball and socket
    (B) Pivot
    (C) Saddle
    (D) Hinge

GO ON TO THE NEXT PAGE

Refer to the following radiograph for Questions 61 and 62:

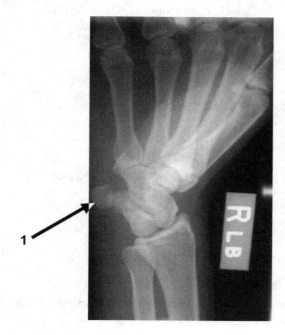

61.

What is the projection of the wrist being demonstrated here?

(A) PA oblique, lateral rotation

(B) AP oblique, medial rotation

(C) Radial deviation

(D) Ulna deviation

62. Which structure is identified by Arrow 1?

(A) Scaphoid

(B) Lunate

(C) Capitate

(D) Pisiform

63. What is the position of the fingers for a PA wrist?

(A) Fully extended

(B) Flexed

(C) Oblique

(D) Dorsiflexed

64. What is the central ray angle for an AP projection of the knee when the patient's ASIS measures 26 cm from the tabletop?

(A) 0

(B) 3 to 5° caudad

(C) 3 to 5° cephalad

(D) 10° cephalad

65. How must the fingers be to demonstrate the interphalangeal joints of the hand in the oblique position?

(A) Touching the image receptor

(B) Parallel to the image receptor

(C) Flexed

(D) Hyperextended

66. For the lateral forearm projection, the elbow must be flexed how many degrees?

(A) 0°

(B) 20°

(C) 45°

(D) 90°

67. For digits 2 to 5, which joint is used as the centering point?

(A) DIP

(B) PIP

(C) MCP

(D) CMC

68. Which view of the ankle demonstrates the talofibular joint space in profile?

(A) AP

(B) AP, internal rotation 15°

(C) AP, internal rotation 45°

(D) Lateral

GO ON TO THE NEXT PAGE

69. Which projection BEST demonstrates possible cartilage degeneration of the knees?

   (A) AP
   (B) AP, weight-bearing
   (C) PA axial, intercondylar fossa
   (D) Lateral

70. What is the central ray angle for demonstration of the radial head utilizing the axial trauma projection (Coyle)?

   (A) 45° toward shoulder
   (B) 45° toward wrist
   (C) 20° toward shoulder
   (D) 20° toward wrist

Other

1. The introduction of contrast medium for myelography can be accomplished at which level?

   (A) T11–T12
   (B) L1–L2
   (C) L3–L4
   (D) L5–S1

2. Which is the contrast-media study of synovial joints and related soft-tissue structures?

   (A) Arthrography
   (B) Venography
   (C) Sialography
   (D) Orthoroentgenography

3. The femoral vein is used for catheterization during which of the following venogram studies?

   1. Inferior venacavogram
   2. Renal venogram
   3. Lower limb venogram

   (A) 1 only
   (B) 1 and 2 only
   (C) 2 and 3 only
   (D) 1, 2, and 3

4. For a myelogram, the contrast is injected into which area of the spinal cord?

   (A) Pia mater
   (B) Arachnoid space
   (C) Subarachnoid space
   (D) Conus medullaris

5. Which of the following would visualize the lodging of an embolus in a blood vessel?

   (A Venogram
   (B) Arthrogram
   (C) Sialogram
   (D) Myelogram

6. For a venogram of the lower extremities, what is the rotation of the lower legs?

   (A) Internal rotation, 10°
   (B) External rotation, 10°
   (C) Internal rotation, 30°
   (D) External rotation, 30°

7. A myelogram is contraindicated for which of the following?

   1. Blood in cerebrospinal fluid
   2. Inflammation of the arachnoid membrane
   3. Increased intracranial pressure

   (A) 3 only
   (B) 1 and 2 only
   (C) 2 and 3 only
   (D) 1, 2, and 3

GO ON TO THE NEXT PAGE

Answers and Explanations

Thorax

1. The correct answer is (B).

The mediastinum contains all thoracic organs except the lungs. The thymus gland (A), a structure associated with the immune system, is very prominent during infancy. It reaches its maximum size during puberty, and decreases in size, almost disappearing, as an adult. The proximal esophagus (D) is located posterior to the trachea (C) within the mediastinum.

2. The correct answer is (C).

The right lung has three lobes—superior (upper), middle, and inferior (lower)—separated by two fissures. The left lung has two lobes—the superior (upper) and inferior (lower)—separated by an oblique fissure.

3. The correct answer is (D).

To separate the vertebrae and sternum, one needs to rotate the body from the prone position or to angle the central ray medially. The depth of the chest determines the required angulation. The range is 15 to 20° of obliquity (15° for thicker thorax and 20° for thinner). Angulation of the body or central ray that projects the sternum to the left of the thoracic vertebrae, as with the RAO body position, will superimpose it over the homogeneous density of the heart, where it is better visualized.

4. The correct answer is (B).

The diaphragm is the muscle of respiration. In the recumbent position, gravitational force causes the abdominal viscera and diaphragm to move superiorly; it compresses the thoracic viscera, which prevents full expansion of the lungs.

5. The correct answer is (D).

Inspiration and expiration radiographs demonstrate pneumothorax (gas or air in the pleural cavity), occasional presence of a foreign body, and atelectasis (absence of air).

6. The correct answer is (C).

To include both lungs from apices to costophrenic angles, the centering point is generally at the level of T7.

7. The correct answer is (A).

Emphysema is a condition in which the lung bases present a flattened appearance rather than the typical dome shape. Areas of increased blackening or radiolucency also appear, caused by the destruction of distal bronchioles and alveoli.

8. The correct answer is (C).

There are three main parts to the pharynx: nasopharynx (posterior to the two nasal cavities), oropharynx (behind mouth), and laryngopharynx (located inferior to epiglottis).

9. The correct answer is (D).

For anterior obliques, the side of interest is generally the side farthest from the image receptor. Thus, the RAO will best visualize the left lung whereas the LAO will best visualize the right. For a routine study, these will be 45° obliques. Certain positions for studies of the heart require an LAO with an increased rotation to 60°. Less rotation (15 to 20°) may be requested for better visualization of possible pulmonary disease.

10. The correct answer is (A).

If the patient is too weak to stand and lean back for an upright AP lordotic, you can take an AP semiaxial projection with the patient supine. The patient's shoulders are rolled forward to move scapulae laterally; the central ray is directed 15 to 20° cephalad, to midsternum.

11. The correct answer is (A).

12. The correct answer is (C).

13. The correct answer is (D).

The dense area being identified is the area of the hilum. The hilum, also known as the root region, is the depression that accommodates the bronchi, pulmonary blood vessels, lymph vessels, and nerves. The pleura (D) is a double-walled serous membrane sac in which each lung is enclosed.

14. The correct answer is (B).

The first 10 thoracic vertebrae have facets on their transverse processes that articulate with the tubercles of ribs 1 to 10. These articulations are termed costotransverse joints. The only articulation for ribs 11 and 12 is at their costovertebral joints.

15. The correct answer is (B).

For the PA oblique projection, the affected side is positioned 45° away from the image receptor. So the LAO position demonstrates right-side ribs. Respiration should be suspended at the end of full inspiration for ribs above the diaphragm and on full expiration for ribs below the diaphragm.

16. The correct answer is (B).

The epiglottis is located on top of the larynx. It covers the larynx as one swallows to prevent food and fluids from entering the trachea instead of the esophagus. The cricoid cartilage (C) is a ring of cartilage that forms the inferior margin of the larynx. The thyroid cartilage (D) is the most prominent cartilage of the larynx, located approximately at the level of C5.

17. The correct answer is (A).

Arrow 1 identifies the left primary bronchus, Arrow 2 identifies the alveoli, Arrow 3 identifies the pleura, Arrow 4 identifies the carina, and Arrow 5 identifies the right primary bronchus.

18. The correct answer is (D).

The right primary bronchus is wider, shorter, and more vertical than the left bronchus (A); foreign bodies entering the airway are more likely to pass into and possibly lodge on this side.

19. The correct answer is (C).

Pleural effusion is a condition of abnormal accumulation of fluid in the pleural cavity. Atelectasis (A) is when all or a portion of a lung collapses. Pneumothorax (B) is an accumulation of air in the pleural space, causing partial or complete collapse of a lung. With bronchitis (D), an acute or chronic condition, excessive mucus is secreted into the bronchi, creating cough and shortness of breath.

20. The correct answer is (C).

The carina is a ridge of the lowest tracheal cartilage, where it divides into right and left bronchi. The position of the carina is at the lower level of the division into the right and left primary bronchi. This is at the approximate level of T5 and is used as a reference point for CT of the thorax.

Abdomen and GI Studies

1. The correct answer is (C).

The cecum (A) is a portion of the large intestine below the ileocecal valve, to which the appendix is attached. The duodenum (B) is the first part of the small intestine, also the widest and the shortest. The first two-fifths following the duodenum is the jejunum (D), and the remaining three-fifths of the small intestine is called the ileum.

2. The correct answer is (D).

Digestion and absorption of food occur within the small intestine. The mucosa of the small intestine contains fingerlike projections called villi, which aid in the process.

3. The correct answer is (C).

The right lateral decubitus position demonstrates an AP or PA projection of the contrast-filled colon. This position best demonstrates the "up" medial side of the ascending colon and the lateral side of the descending colon, when the colon is inflated with air.

4. The correct answer is (A).

An intussusception occurs when a segment of bowel, constricted by peristalsis, telescopes into a distal segment and is driven further into the distal bowel by peristalsis. A volvulus (B) is a twisting of a bowel loop. (C) Paralytic ileus or adynamic ileus is a failure of normal peristalsis. Varicose veins (D) are abnormally lengthened, dilated, and superficial veins; those in the esophagus are referred to as esophageal varices.

5. The correct answer is (B).

In the prone or anterior oblique position, the fundus is at its highest portion, causing the air to fill this part of the stomach during a double-contrast examination.

6. The correct answer is (D).

When the patient is in the prone position, the central ray should be angled 30 to 40° caudad to demonstrate the rectosigmoid area with less superimposition than the PA projection due to the angulation of the central ray.

7. The correct answer is (D).

The sigmoid colon is one of four parts of the colon (ascending, descending, and transverse are the other three). These are all a portion of the large intestine, which has four major parts: cecum, colon, rectum, and anal canal.

8. The correct answer is (C).

For the small bowel series, typically 2 cups of barium is ingested by the patient. For the enteroclysis procedure, the patient is intubated under fluoroscopic control with a special enteroclysis catheter that passes through the stomach into the duodenum. For the intubation method, a nasogastric tube is passed through the patient's nose, through the esophagus, stomach, and duodenum, and into the jejunum.

9. The correct answer is (D).

A lateral projection shows the anterior and posterior aspects of the stomach, the pyloric canal, and the duodenal bulb.

10. The correct answer is (C).

The stomach's right border is marked by the lesser curvature, which begins at the esophagogastric junction and is a concave curve ending at the pylorus. The stomach's left and inferior borders are marked by the greater curvature, which begins at the sharp angle of the esophagogastric junction around the fundus (B), and then the convex curvature of the body down to the pylorus.

11. The correct answer is (A).

The esophagus joins the stomach at the esophagogastric junction through an opening called the cardiac orifice. The muscles that control the cardiac orifice are called the cardiac sphincter.

12. The correct answer is (B).

For the PA oblique projection RAO, the stomach and entire duodenal loop is presented. This gives the best image of the pyloric canal and the duodenal bulb in sthenic patients. Gastric peristalsis is generally more active with the patient in the RAO position.

13. The correct answer is (A).

A sliding hiatal hernia may produce a radiographic sign called Schatzki's ring, a ringlike constriction at the distal esophagus caused by a weakening of the esophageal sphincter located between the terminal esophagus and the diaphragm.

14. The correct answer is (B).

The cecum is the widest portion of the large intestine and moves about fairly freely in the right lower quadrant.

15. The correct answer is (B).

The terminal portion of the ileum, the ileocecal valve, and the cecum of the large intestine are best shown on a spot film of this area. A spot film such as this, using a compression cone, is usually taken at the ileocecal valve area at the end of a small bowel series to best visualize this region.

16. The correct answer is (D).

The muscular portion of the intestinal wall of the large intestine contains three external bands of muscle fibers to form taeniae coli, which pull the large intestine into pouches. Each of these pouches is termed a haustrum. So an identifying characteristic of the large bowel is the presence of multiple haustra.

17. The correct answer is (B).

During a double-contrast barium enema, when a person is supine, air rises to fill the most anterior structures: the transverse colon and loops of sigmoid colon. The barium sinks to fill primarily the ascending, descending, and parts of the sigmoid colon.

18. The correct answer is (B).

The left colic flexure should be seen without superimposition in the LAO of 35 to 45° rotation. It is also seen in the RPO position.

19. The correct answer is (C).

Due to evidence in the radiograph of a horizontal air-fluid line, we can ascertain that the image was obtained with the patient in the erect position.

20. The correct answer is (D).

The decubitus position—specifically, the left lateral decubitus position—will best demonstrate air and fluid levels within the abdominal cavity, since the density of the liver provides good contrast for visualization of free air. This projection is especially helpful in assessing free air in the abdomen when an upright position is not possible.

21. The correct answer is (C).

The centering for an AP supine abdomen is to the midsagittal plane at the level of the iliac crests. The iliac crests are at the level of L4–5 interspace.

22. The correct answer is (B).

Because there is no air being introduced into the large intestine as with the double-contrast barium enema, the decubitus images (demonstrating air-fluid) are not taken.

23. The correct answer is (A).

During a single-contrast examination of the stomach, the head of the table is lowered 25 to 30° for demonstration of a hiatal hernia, placing the patient in Trendelenberg.

24. The correct answer is (D).

The PA, post-evacuation, demonstrates the mucosal pattern of the large intestine with residual contrast media for demonstrating small polyps and defects.

25. The correct answer is (B).

The esophagram, or barium swallow, studies the form and function of the swallowing aspect of the pharynx and esophagus. The upper gastrointestinal series studies the distal esophagus, stomach, and duodenum.

KAPLAN

26. The correct answer is (A).

The alimentary canal begins at the oral cavity; continues as the pharynx, then esophagus, stomach (B), small intestine (C), and large intestine (D).

27. The correct answer is (A).

The endoscopic retrograde cholangiopancreatography procedure (ERCP) includes the endoscopic insertion of the catheter or injection cannula into the common bile duct or main pancreatic duct under fluoroscopic control, followed by retrograde injection of contrast media into the biliary ducts. The endoscope is visible in the radiograph included here.

28. The correct answer is (A).

To examine the biliary and main pancreatic ducts, one uses the endoscopic retrograde cholangio-pancreatography procedure (ERCP).

29. The correct answer is (A).

For the RAO position, the esophagus should be visualized between the vertebral column and heart. (RAO provides more visibility of pertinent anatomy than does the LAO for an oblique esophagus.)

30. The correct answer is (C).

The patient is rotated between 30 and 60° for obliques of the stomach. The sthenic type is rotated 45°; the hypersthenic patient, 60°; and the asthenic patient, 30°.

31. The correct answer is (B).

Peristalsis is a wavelike series of involuntary muscular contractions propelling solid and semisolid materials through the alimentary canal. Deglutition (A) is the act of swallowing. Mastication (D) is the chewing movement as part of mechanical digestion.

Urological Studies

1. The correct answer is (A).

The patient is in the modified lithotomy position for retrograde urography. The patient is placed on the cystoscopic table with knees flexed over the stirrups of the adjustable leg supports.

2. The correct answer is (C).

The post-void, upright position may demonstrate an enlarged prostate or prolapse of the bladder. The erect position also demonstrates nephroptosis (position change of the kidneys).

3. The correct answer is (D).

Horseshoe kidney occurs when the lower poles of the kidneys are joined across the midline by a band of soft tissues. Kidney function is generally unimpaired with this condition. Hydronephrosis (A) is an obstructive disease of the urinary system that causes a dilation, possibly leading to intrarenal pressure causing parenchymal atrophy. Polycystic kidney disease (B) is a congenital disorder presenting tiny cysts that enlarge and destroy normal tissue. Nephrosclerosis (C), thickening of the small vessels of the kidney, causes atrophy of the renal parenchyma over time.

4. The correct answer is (A).

For voiding cystourethrography, the male is best examined in a 30° right posterior oblique position. The female is usually examined in the AP or slight oblique position.

5. The correct answer is (A).

Radiographs taken 1 minute after the start of injection are called nephrograms. The renal parenchyma or functional portion of the kidney consists of many thousands of nephrons. Because individual nephrons are microscopic, the nephron phase is a blush of the entire kidney substance. The blush results from contrast medium being dispersed throughout the many nephrons but not into the collecting tubules as yet.

6. The correct answer is (D).

There are three common points of constriction of the ureter where a stone may become lodged. The first point is the ureteropelvic junction (where the renal pelvis empties into the ureter). The second point is the pelvic brim (iliac blood vessels cross over ureters). The third is the area where the ureters join the bladder, posteriorly, termed the ureterovesical junction.

7. The correct answer is (D).

For an AP oblique projection of the bladder (RPO, LPO), rotate the patient 40 to 60°, according to the preference of the examining physician. Oblique projections demonstrate the bladder filled with contrast. If reflux is present, the distal ureters are also visualized.

8. The correct answer is (D).

The conditions that exist that would contraindicate ureteric compression are ureteric stones, abdominal mass, abdominal aortic aneurysm, recent abdominal surgery, severe abdominal pain, and acute abdominal trauma.

9. The correct answer is (D).

The obliques for the kidneys are performed at 30° so as to place the kidney on the elevated side in profile or parallel to the image receptor. As a result, the RPO best demonstrates the left kidney and the LPO best demonstrates the right.

10. The correct answer is (B).

The central ray is angled 10 to 15° caudad to enter 2 inches above the upper border of the pubic symphysis. When the bladder neck and proximal urethra are the main areas of interest, a 5° caudal angulation is sufficient to project the pubic bones below them.

11. The correct answer is (A).

The intravenous urography (IVU) is the most common radiographic exam of the urinary system. The IVU is a true function test in that the contrast medium molecules are rapidly removed from the bloodstream and excreted completely by the normal kidney.

12. The correct answer is (D).

The voiding cystourethrogram (VCU) provides a study of the urethra and evaluates the patient's ability to urinate; therefore, it is a functional study of the bladder and urethra. Retrograde urography (B) is a nonfunctional exam of the urinary system.

13. The correct answer is (C).

The renal pelvis lies within the hilum, and its tapering lower part passes through the hilum to be continuous with the ureter.

14. The correct answer is (A).

The calyces are stems arising at the sides of the papilla of each renal pyramid. Each calyx encloses one or more papillae. The beginning branches are called the minor calyces, and they unite to form two or three larger tubes called the major calyces. The major calyces unite to form the expanded, funnel-shaped renal pelvis (D).

15. The correct answer is (B).

The renal medulla is composed mainly of the collecting tubules that give it a striated appearance, and consists of 8 to 15 cone-shaped segments called renal pyramids. The renal sinus (1) is a fat-filled space surrounding the renal pelvis (3) and vessels.

Spine and Pelvis

1. The correct answer is (A).

Each hipbone consists of three divisions: ilium (B), ischium (C), and pubis (D). These three bones join together to form the acetabulum, the socket that receives the head of the femur.

2. The correct answer is (B).

The cross-table lateral hip is a common projection for patients who cannot move or rotate the affected leg for the frog-leg lateral. The image receptor is placed parallel to the femoral neck and the central ray is directed perpendicular to both.

3. The correct answer is (D).

The left intervertebral foramina are being visualized on this radiograph. The central ray is directed 15° caudad to C4 for anterior obliques (foramina closest to IR demonstrated), and 15° cephalad for posterior obliques (foramina farthest from IR demonstrated). If it is a PA oblique projection, it must be the LAO body position.

4. The correct answer is (C).

For obliques of the cervical spine, rotate the patient 45° to visualize the intervertebral foramina.

5. The correct answer is (B).

The PA projection of the lumbar spine places the intervertebral disk spaces at an angle closely paralleling the divergence of the beam of radiation. This projection also reduces the dose to the patient. An AP projection utilizes an extended leg position that accentuates the lordotic curve, resulting in distortion of the bodies and poor delineation of the intervertebral disk spaces. This curve can be reduced by flexing the patient's hips and knees enough to place the back in contact with the radiographic table.

6. The correct answer is (A).

For demonstration of the lumbar zygapophyseal joints, rotate the patient 45°. RPO and LPO body positions demonstrate the downside; LAO and RAO demonstrate the upside.

7. The correct answer is (B).

The Jefferson fracture occurs as a result of axial loading, such as landing on one's head. The anterior and posterior arches of C1 are fractured as the skull slams onto the ring. The open-mouth projection and lateral cervical spine projections will demonstrate this. Clay shoveler's fracture (A) results from hyperflexion of the neck resulting in avulsion fracture of the spinous process of C6–T1. Hangman's fracture (C) extends through the pedicles of C2 when the neck is subject to extreme hyperextension.

8. The correct answer is (B).

Spondylolysis is an acquired bony defect occurring in the pars interarticularis, the area of the lamina between the two articular processes. The defect may occur on one or both sides of the vertebra, resulting in a condition termed spondylolisthesis.

9. The correct answer is (C).

Both right and left obliques are taken for comparison with the patient in a 45° posterior oblique. When evaluating the downside acetabulum, the anterior rim of the acetabulum and the posterior ilioischial column are demonstrated. When centered to the upside acetabulum, the posterior rim of the acetabulum and the anterior ilioischial column are demonstrated.

10. The correct answer is (D).

The cervical and lumbar curves, which are convex anteriorly, are called lordotic curves. The thoracic and pelvic curves are concave anteriorly and are called kyphotic curves. The thoracic and pelvic curves are also called primary curves because they are present at birth. The cervical and lumbar curves are called secondary or compensatory curves because they develop after birth.

11. The correct answer is (C).

For visualization of the sacroiliac joints with an AP oblique projection, the side under examination should be elevated approximately 25 to 30°. The side being examined is farther from the image receptor. Use the LPO position to demonstrate the right joint and the RPO position to show the left joint.

12. The correct answer is (C).

The head and neck of the femur is angled 15 to 20° anteriorly in relationship to the body of the femur. Therefore, the femur and leg must be rotated 15 to 20° internally to place the femoral neck parallel to the image receptor for a true AP projection of the proximal femur. If a patient is unable to rotate the lower extremity due to trauma, the AP will be obtained "as is."

13. The correct answer is (B).

A good 45° oblique of the lumbar spine projects the various structures in a way that a "Scotty dog" seems to appear. The neck is one pars interarticularis, the ear of the dog is one superior articular process, the eye is formed by one pedicle, one transverse process forms the nose, and the front legs are formed by one inferior articular process.

14. The correct answer is (D).

The laminae of the lumbar vertebrae form a bridge between the transverse processes, lateral masses, and spinous process. The portion of each lamina between the superior and inferior articular processes is the pars interarticularis. The pars interarticularis is demonstrated radiographically on the oblique lumbar spine image.

15. The correct answer is (C).

Spondylolisthesis involves forward movement of one vertebra in relation to another. It is commonly due to a developmental defect of the pars interarticularis or may result from spondylolysis or severe osteoarthritis. It is most common at L5–S1, but also occurs at L4–L5. Spondylolysis (C) is a separation of the pars interarticularis, but there is no forward movement of the vertebra. Ankylosing spondylitis (A) is an inflammatory condition that usually begins in the sacroiliac joints and progresses up the vertebral column. Spina bifida (D) is a congenital condition in which the posterior aspects of the vertebrae fail to develop, exposing part of the spinal cord.

16. The correct answer is (C).

In the case of suspected hip fracture, the unilateral frog-leg should not be performed on the patient. Instead, to provide a lateral view, the cross-table lateral or the modified axiolateral (Clements-Nakayama) could be used.

17. The correct answer is (A).

The AP bilateral frog-leg projection (modified Cleaves) is useful for demonstration of developmental dysplasia of hip (DDH), also known as congenital hip dislocation (CHD). This is performed frequently for periodic follow-up exams on younger patients.

18. The correct answer is (A).

For the lateral L5–S1 cone-down, if there is not enough waist support to prevent sag of the lumbar vertebrae, an angle of 5 to 8° caudad to be parallel to the interiliac plane (imaginary line between iliac crests) opens the joint space.

19. The correct answer is (D).

The sacrum is formed by the fusion of five sacral vertebral segments into a curved, triangular bone.

20. The correct answer is (D).

The sacrum and coccyx are commonly imaged together. To obtain the laterals with one exposure, the central ray is directed perpendicular to a point 3-4 inches posterior to the ASIS (anterior superior iliac spine).

21. The correct answer is (B).

The lamina forms a bridge between the transverse processes, lateral masses, and spinous process.

22. The correct answer is (A).

The intervertebral foramina are spaces or openings between the pedicles when two vertebrae are stacked on each other. Along the upper surface of each pedicle is a half-moon-shaped area (the superior vertebral notch); along the lower surface of each pedicle is another half-moon-shaped area (the inferior vertebral notch). Between every two vertebrae, therefore, are two intervertebral foramina, one on each side.

23. The correct answer is (C).

The transverse processes of lumbar vertebrae are smaller than those of the thoracic vertebrae. The superior three pairs are directed almost exactly laterally, whereas the inferior two pair are included slightly superiorly.

24. The correct answer is (A).

On the lumbar vertebrae, the spinous processes are large, thick, and blunt, and they have an almost horizontal projection posteriorly. The palpable tip of each spinous process corresponds in position with the interspace below the vertebra from which it projects.

25. The correct answer is (B).

For an AP coccyx with the patient supine, the central ray is directed 10° caudad and enters a point 2 inches superior to the pubic symphysis. With the patient prone, the central ray will be angled 10° cephalad.

26. The correct answer is (B).

The lateral projection of the thoracic spine demonstrates lateral thoracic bodies and their interspaces, the intervertebral foramina, and the lower spinous processes.

27. The correct answer is (D).

For the PA (Judd) for visualization of the dens, the chin rests on the table top and is extended to bring the MML as nearly perpendicular to the table as possible. This will demonstrate the dens and other structures of C1–C2 within the foramen magnum.

28. The correct answer is (C).

To demonstrate the L5–S1 interspace and the sacroiliac joints, the central ray is directed 30° cephalad for males and 35° cephalad for females to the level of the ASIS.

29. The correct answer is (A).

The greater trochanter is most prominent laterally and more easily palpated when the lower leg is medially rotated. This point is in the same horizontal plane as the pubic symphysis.

30. The correct answer is (C).

At the junction of the pedicle and lamina, behind the transverse process, are the cervical articular processes. Between the superior and articular processes is a short column, or pillar, of bone that is highly supportive. This column of bone is called the articular pillar or lateral mass when referring to C1.

31. The correct answer is (D).

The inverted "V" is the spinous process of C2.

32. The correct answer is (A).

Unlike the other zygapophyseal joints of the cervical spine, those between C1 and C2 are visualized only on a true AP projection (open-mouth). The second through seventh cervical vertebrae are located at right angles to the midsagittal plane and are visualized only in a true lateral position.

33. The correct answer is (B).

For the open-mouth projection of the cervical spine the patient opens the mouth as wide as possible, and then the head is adjusted so that a line from the lower edge of the upper incisors to the tip of the mastoid process (occlusal plane) is perpendicular to the image receptor.

Cranium

1. The correct answer is (C).

The skull has 22 bones, consisting of 14 facial bones and 8 cranial bones.

2. The correct answer is (A).

The crista galli arises from the cribriform plate of the ethmoid bone.

3. The correct answer is (A).

The Waters method best demonstrates the maxillary sinuses. The PA axial (Caldwell) best demonstrates the frontal and anterior ethmoid sinuses. The SMV (C) demonstrates the ethmoidal and sphenoidal sinuses. The lateral view (D) demonstrates all of the sinuses, but the sphenoidal sinus is of primary importance.

4. The correct answer is (A).

The frontal bone is best demonstrated in a PA projection of the skull.

5. The correct answer is (D).

The sella turcica is a structure that houses the pituitary gland and is a portion of the sphenoid bone.

6. The correct answer is (D).

The temporal bone holds the organs of hearing within the petrous portion, the densest area of bone in the cranium.

7. The correct answer is (B).

The occipital bone has a large aperture, the foramen magnum, through which the inferior portion of the medulla oblongata passes as it exits the cranial cavity and joins the spinal cord.

8. The correct answer is (A).

For demonstration of the TMJ closest to the image receptor, the face must be rotated toward the image receptor 15° and the central ray will be directed 15° caudad. Closed-mouth image demonstrates the condyle within the mandibular fossa; in open-mouth, the condyle moves to the anterior margin of the mandibular fossa.

9. The correct answer is (B).

The central ray is directed to exit the nasion at an angle of 15° caudad.

10. The correct answer is (D).

The zygomatic arches will be demonstrated in the parietoacanthial (Waters), submentovertical, and AP axial (Towne).

11. The correct answer is (D).

The submentovertical projection demonstrates advanced bony pathology of the inner temporal bone structures (skull base) and basal skull fractures are demonstrated.

12. The correct answer is (C).

The figure describes positioning for the PA axial Haas method. The occipital bone is best demonstrated with the PA axial Haas method of the skull.

13. The correct answer is (B).

When the Haas method for demonstration of the occipital bone cannot be obtained, the alternative is to perform the AP axial (Towne). For the AP axial (Towne), the central ray is directed 30° caudad when the OML is perpendicular to the plane of the image receptor. If the patient is unable to line up the OML, then the IOML can be used and the central ray will be directed 37° caudad.

14. The correct answer is (D).

For an axiolateral oblique of the mandible from the lateral position, when the head is rotated 45° the mentum is visualized, 30° the body, 15° general survey, and 0° the ramus.

15. The correct answer is (A).

The coronoid process of the mandible is the anterior process—it must not be confused with the coronoid process of the proximal ulna of the forearm or the coracoid process (B)—of the scapula. The posterior process of the upper ramus is termed the condyloid process (C).

16. The correct answer is (C).

The condyle of the mandible articulates with the mandibular fossa of the temporal bone.

17. The correct answer is (A).

For the PA projection, with the OML perpendicular to the image receptor, the orbits are filled by the margins of the petrous pyramids. When the central ray is angled 15° caudad to the nasion, the petrous ridges are projected into the lower third of the orbits.

18. The correct answer is (D).

The two bones of the face that are not paired are the mandible and vomer. There are six pairs of 14 facial bones, which include maxillae, zygomatic, palatine, nasal, lacrimal, and inferior nasal conchae.

19. The correct answer is (D).

A tripod fracture is caused by a direct blow to the cheek. As a result, the zygoma will fracture in three places: the orbital process, the maxillary process, and the arch.

20. The correct answer is (C).

The OML forms a 37° angle to the plane of the image receptor for the parietoacanthial (Waters). Fractures (particularly blowout, tripod, and LeFort fractures) are shown.

21. The correct answer is (A).

With a 25° cephalad angle of the central ray in the PA projection, the TMJ region and heads of condyles are visible through the mastoid processes; the PA axial best demonstrates the proximal rami and condyloid processes.

22. The correct answer is (B).

The sphenoid sinuses are visualized through the open mouth for the open-mouth Waters projection.

23. The correct answer is (A).

The interpupillary line is perpendicular to the plane of the image receptor, ensuring no tilt of the head. The IOML is perpendicular to the front edge of the image receptor but is parallel to the long axis of the image receptor.

24. The correct answer is (B).

The lateral projection demonstrates the sphenoid sinuses posterior to and without superimposition of the ethmoid sinuses. The submentovertical projection demonstrates the sphenoid sinuses anterior to the foramen magnum. With the PA (Caldwell) projection, the sphenoid sinuses are not demonstrated specifically, because they are located directly posterior to the ethmoid sinuses.

Extremities

1. The correct answer is (B).

The coracoid process can be felt just distal and slightly medial to the acromioclavicular articulation. It rises from the base of the scapular notch to the superior portion of the neck of the scapula. The acromion (Arrow 4) is a flattened end of the scapular spine.

2. The correct answer is (A).

The subscapular fossa is on the costal (anterior) surface of the scapula. It is filled almost entirely by the attachment of the subscapularis muscle. On the dorsal surface of the scapula is the scapular spine; the supraspinous fossa is above the spine and the portion below the spine is the infraspinous fossa.

3. The correct answer is (D).

The lateral (axillary) border extends from the glenoid cavity to the inferior angle of the scapula. The medial (vertebral) border runs parallel with the vertebral column. The superior border extends from the superior angle to the coracoid process and scapular notch.

4. The correct answer is (B).

The patient's leg is rotated medially until the plantar surface of the foot forms an angle of 30° to the plane of the image receptor. If the angle of the foot is increased more than that, the lateral cuneiform tends to be thrown over the other cuneiforms.

5. The correct answer is (C).

For an AP projection of the forearm, the patient is seated at the end of the table with the hand and arm supinated (fully extended, palm up).

6. The correct answer is (D).

The lateral projection of the elbow, flexion of 90°, demonstrates the olecranon process in profile. The elbow fat pads are also the least compressed in this position.

7. The correct answer is (C).

For the plantodorsal (axial) projection of the calcaneus, the central ray is directed at a cephalic angle of 40° to the long axis of the foot. The central ray enters about the base of the third (fifth) metatarsal, which demonstrates the calcaneus and subtalar joint.

8. The correct answer is (A).

The thumb has only two phalanges, so there is only one interphalangeal (IP) joint between them. The second through fifth digits each have three phalanges; therefore, they have two interphalangeal joints each (one proximal, one distal).

9. The correct answer is (D).

Both AP and lateral weight-bearing projections of the foot are useful in demonstrating the bones of the feet to show the condition of the longitudinal arches under the full weight of the body. Laterals of both feet are usually taken for comparison.

10. The correct answer is (C).

An AP axial projection of 15° posteriorly will better demonstrate the interphalangeal joint spaces. Because of the natural curve of the toes, the interphalangeal joint spaces are not best demonstrated on the AP projection with no angle.

11. The correct answer is (A).

For demonstration of the ankle mortise, the patient will rotate the entire leg and foot internally 15 to 20° until the intermalleolar plane is parallel with the image receptor.

12. The correct answer is (B).

The talus occupies the most superior portion of the foot. It is the second largest tarsal bone (first is calcaneus). It articulates with four other bones: the tibia, fibula, calcaneus, and navicular. The superior surface, the trochlear surface, articulates with the tibia.

13. The correct answer is (B).

The fibula articulates with the tibia at both its distal and proximal ends. The distal tibiofibular joint is a fibrous syndesmosis joint allowing slight movement.

14. The correct answer is (A).

The medial malleolus is a large process on the distal end of the tibia. The lateral malleolus (Arrow 3) is the enlarged distal end of the fibula. The medial and lateral condyles (C) and (D) are two prominent processes at the proximal end of the tibia.

15. The correct answer is (A).

The proximal row of carpal bones from lateral to medial is scaphoid, lunate, triquetrum, and pisiform. The distal row, from lateral to medial, is trapezium, trapezoid, capitate, and hamate.

16. The correct answer is (D).

For a PA projection of the hand, the central ray is directed to the third metacarpophalangeal joint (MCP).

17. The correct answer is (D).

AP and lateral projections of the knee best demonstrate Osgood-Schlatter disease, which is a fragmentation and/or detachment of the tibial tuberosity by the patellar tendon (avulsion of the tibial tuberosity).

18. The correct answer is (A).

A PA projection of the hand demonstrates an oblique projection of the first digit.

19. The correct answer is (D).

For an AP axial projection of the clavicle, the central ray is directed 15 to 30° cephalad to mid-clavicle. Thin (asthenic) patients require 10 to 15° more angle than those with thick shoulders and chest (hypersthenic).

20. The correct answer is (C).

The proximal end of the femurs consists of two large processes: the greater trochanter and the lesser trochanter. The greater trochanter is at the superolateral part of the femoral body, and the lesser trochanter is at the posteromedial part.

21. The correct answer is (D).

The smooth, rounded head of the femur is at the proximal end and is connected to the femoral body by a pyramid-shaped neck; it is received into the acetabular cavity of the hip bone.

22. The correct answer is (C).

Most primary centers of bone formation or ossification, such as those involving the midshaft area of long bones, appear before birth. These primary centers become the diaphysis (shaft or body) of long bones. Each secondary center of ossification involves the ends of long bones and is termed an epiphysis (A). The space between the diaphysis and the epiphysis is made up of cartilage and is termed an epiphyseal plate (B). Full maturity is at about 25 years of age.

23. The correct answer is (D).

The transthoracic lateral projection is used when trauma exists and the arm cannot be rotated or abducted because of an injury. For the inferosuperior axial (A), the patient must abduct the arm from the body as much as possible.

24. The correct answer is (B).

Two sets of bilateral acromioclavicular (AC) joints are taken in the same position, one without weights and one stress view with weights (after fracture has been ruled out). AC joint separation is demonstrated. A widening of one joint space, as compared with the other view with weights, usually indicates an AC joint separation.

25. The correct answer is (A).

When the image receptor and wrist are placed horizontally, the central ray can be directed 20° toward the elbow (proximally).

26. The correct answer is (C).

For the scapular Y position, the patient is rotated so that the midcoronal plane forms an angle of 45 to 60° to the image receptor. The flat surface of the scapula is perpendicular to the image receptor. The projection is useful in the evaluation of suspected shoulder dislocations.

27. The correct answer is (C).

For an AP projection of the shoulder (internal, neutral, or external rotation), the central ray is directed to a point 1 inch inferior to the coracoid process.

28. The correct answer is (B).

With the AP humerus, the arm is abducted slightly and the hand is supinated (places epicondyles parallel with plane of image receptor); this will demonstrate the humeral head and greater tubercle in profile on the radiograph.

29. The correct answer is (A).

On the medial proximal aspect of the calcaneus is a large prominent bony process called the sustentaculum tali, which acts as a support for the talus.

30. The correct answer is (D).

The lateral—in either extension or flexion—is utilized for localization of foreign bodies of the hand and fingers and also demonstrates the anterior or posterior displaced fractures of the metacarpals.

31. The correct answer is (B).

For a lateral knee radiograph, rotate the leg and knee into true lateral position with the knee flexed 20 to 30°. Additional flexion will tighten muscles and tendons that may obscure diagnostic information at the joint space.

32. The correct answer is (B).

On a true lateral of the knee, the patellofemoral and femorotibial joint spaces are open. The proximal tibiofibular is not seen as open on the lateral due to the slight superimposition of the fibular head on the tibia (medial oblique knee is best demonstration of open proximal tibiofibular joint).

33. The correct answer is (A).

For the lateral knee, the central ray is directed to the knee joint at an angle of 5 to 7° cephalad to prevent the joint space from being obscured by the magnified image of the medial femoral condyle. In the lateral recumbent position, the medial condyle is also slightly inferior to the lateral condyle.

34. The correct answer is (D).

The tangential projection of the toes provides a profile image of the sesamoid bones at the first metatarsophalangeal (MTP) joint.

35. The correct answer is (A).

For the lateral projection of the calcaneus there is no central ray angle; it is perpendicular to the calcaneus, about 1 inch distal to the medial malleolus. This will place the central ray at the subtalar joint.

36. The correct answer is (A).

The bone age is the most commonly used assessment technique for children with either retarded skeletal development or advanced skeletal maturation. An AP radiograph of the left hand and wrist is compared with standards developed to evaluate ossification centers.

37. The correct answer is (C).

For the AP projection of the humerus and the AP shoulder (external rotation), the arm is slightly abducted and then externally rotated (supinated) so that the epicondyles of the elbow are parallel and equidistant from the image receptor.

38. The correct answer is (B).

There are two articulations between the tibia and fibula; one proximal and one distal tibiofibular articulation.

39. The correct answer is (B).

When the patient is placed in a prone position and the leg is flexed 90°, the central ray will be directed about 15 to 20° to the joint space (Settegast).

40. The correct answer is (A).

For an AP thumb, the hand is internally rotated with fingers extended until the posterior surface of the thumb is in contact with the image receptor.

41. The correct answer is (B).

Arrow 3 identifies the coronoid process of the ulna. The coronoid process is seen free of superimposition on the AP oblique projection, medial rotation of the elbow.

42. The correct answer is (D).

The medial epicondyle is superior to the trochlea on the medial aspect of the distal humerus.

43. The correct answer is (D).

The proximal end of the radius is small and presents a flat, disk-like head above a constricted area called the neck. The styloid process of the radius (B) is at the distal end. Arrow 1 identifies the lateral humeral condyle, the capitulum.

44. The correct answer is (B).

For the AP (dorsoplantar) projection of the foot, the central ray is angled 10° posteriorly (toward the heel), which places it perpendicular to the metatarsals, directed to the base of the third metatarsal.

45. The correct answer is (C).

The AP oblique, lateral rotation demonstrates the interspaces between the first and second metatarsals and between the medial and intermediate cuneiforms.

46. The correct answer is (B).

The AP projection, stress method, demonstrates the presence of a ligamentous tear. Rupture of a ligament is demonstrated by widening of the joint space on the side of the injury when, without moving or rotating the lower leg from the supine position, the foot is forcibly turned toward the opposite side.

47. The correct answer is (C).

The AP oblique projection (Grashey) demonstrates the joint space between the humeral head and the glenoid cavity (scapulohumeral joint). It also demonstrates the glenoid cavity in profile.

48. The correct answer is (A).

For a lateral projection of the ankle, the patient is asked to dorsiflex the foot so the plantar surface is at a right angle to the leg (or as far as the patient can tolerate); do not force. This helps to maintain a true lateral position.

49. The correct answer is (C).

A trimalleolar fracture involves the tibia and fibula; there is a fracture to both the medial and lateral malleoli and the posterior tip of the distal tibia.

50. The correct answer is (D).

The radiograph shows the intercondylar fossa (Arrow 2). It appears in profile, open without superimposition by the patella.

51. The correct answer is (C).

With the intercondylar fossa projection, the intercondylar eminences (Arrow 3) of tibia are well visualized and are without superimposition.

52. The correct answer is (D).

The lateral femoral condyle (Arrow 4) and medial femoral condyle (Arrow 1) are apparent on the image of the intercondylar fossa.

53. The correct answer is (A).

For an AP projection of the proximal femur, the leg is internally rotated 15 to 20°. For the distal portion of the femur, the leg is rotated internally 5° for a true AP, as for an AP knee.

54. The correct answer is (A).

For an AP projection of the lower leg (knee and ankle), the leg is adjusted so that the femoral condyles are parallel with the image receptor and the foot is vertical (dorsiflexed).

55. The correct answer is (A).

For a lateral projection of the patella, the patient is asked to flex the affected knee approximately 5 to 10°. Increasing the flexion reduces the patellofemoral joint space. The knee is in the lateral position and the femoral condyles are superimposed; the patella is perpendicular to the image receptor.

56. The correct answer is (B).

When the patient cannot completely extend the elbow, the lateral position (D) is easily performed; however, two AP projections must be obtained to avoid distortion. A separate AP of the distal humerus and proximal forearm is required.

57. The correct answer is (D).

For the lateral projection of the ankle (mediolateral or lateromedial), the fibula is superimposed over the posterior half of the tibia.

58. The correct answer is (B).

For the lateral projection (RAO or LAO) of the scapula, the arm placement is determined by scapular area of interest. When the patient reaches across the front of the chest and grasps the opposite shoulder, this best demonstrates the body of the scapula. If the patient drops the affected arm, flexes the elbow, and places the arm behind the lower back with the arm partially abducted, this best demonstrates the acromion and coracoid processes.

59. The correct answer is (C).

For the carpal canal (tunnel), tangential projection, the patient is asked to hyperextend the wrist (dorsiflex) as far as possible until the long axis of the metacarpals and the fingers are as near vertical as possible, without lifting wrist and forearm from image receptor. The central ray is then angled 25 to 30° to the long axis of the hand.

60. The correct answer is (C).

In the carpometacarpal (CMC) articulations, the first metacarpal and trapezium form a synovial saddle joint; this permits the thumb to oppose the fingers (touch fingertips). The articulations between the second through fifth metacarpals and the trapezoid, capitate, and hamate form synovial gliding joints.

61. The correct answer is (B).

The patient's wrist was positioned in an AP oblique projection that is rotated 45° medially (internally) until it forms a semisupinated position. This position separates the pisiform from the adjacent carpal bones. It also gives a more distinct radiograph of the triquetrum and hamate.

62. The correct answer is (D).

With the AP oblique, medial rotation, the pisiform is separated from the adjacent carpal bones.

63. The correct answer is (B).

For a PA projection of the wrist, the hand is slightly arched at the MCP joints by flexing the digits to place the wrist in close contact with the image receptor.

64. The correct answer is (C).

For an AP projection of the knee, it is suggested that, to determine that the central ray angle is parallel to the tibial plateau for open joint space, one measures distance from ASIS to tabletop to determine central ray angle to be: <19 cm, 3 to 5° caudad; 19 to 24 cm, 0° angle; >24 cm, 3 to 5° cephalad.

65. The correct answer is (B).

To demonstrate the interphalangeal joints of the fingers, the fingers are separated and carefully placed so the hand is supported in a 45° oblique and is parallel to the image receptor.

66. The correct answer is (D).

For a lateral projection of the forearm, the patient is seated next to the radiographic table low enough that the humerus, shoulder joint, and elbow lie in the same plane; the elbow is flexed 90° and the humeral epicondyles are superimposed.

67. The correct answer is (B).

For digits 2 to 5, the central ray is directed to the PIP (proximal interphalangeal joint) of the affected digit.

68. The correct answer is (B).

The AP oblique projection with 15° internal rotation (ankle mortise) demonstrates the talofibular joint space in profile.

69. The correct answer is (B).

The AP weight-bearing projection demonstrates femorotibial joint spaces of the knees for possible cartilage degeneration or other knee joint pathologies. Both knees are included on same exposure for comparison.

70. The correct answer is (A).

To demonstrate the radial head utilizing the trauma axial (Coyle), the patient flexes the elbow 90°, with hand pronated if possible. The central ray is directed 45° toward the shoulder, to mid-elbow joint.

Other

1. The correct answer is (C).

There are generally two locations for the puncture site during myelography: the lumbar (L3–L4) and cervical (C1–C2) areas. The lumbar area is safer, easier on the patient, and most commonly used for the procedure.

2. The correct answer is (A).

Arthrography is a contrast-media study of synovial joints and related soft-tissue structures. The joints include hip, knee, ankle, shoulder, elbow, wrist, and temporomandibular joints. Sialography (C) is the radiographic examination of the salivary glands. Orthoroentgenography (D) is the measurement of long bones.

3. The correct answer is (B).

The femoral vein is access to the renal vein for the renal venogram, and to the common iliac vein or inferior aspect of the inferior vena cava for an inferior venacavogram. Venograms of the lower extremities are usually obtained with contrast medium injected through a needle placed directly into a superficial vein in the foot.

4. The correct answer is (C).

For myelography, contrast is injected into the subarachnoid space by spinal puncture.

5. The correct answer is (A).

A venogram visualizes the lodging of an embolus in a blood vessel.

6. The correct answer is (C).

For venograms of the lower extremities without fluoroscopy, usually AP projections are obtained with the leg internally rotated 30° to include the entire area of interest.

7. The correct answer is (D).

Myelography is contraindicated in the following situations: when there is blood in the cerebrospinal fluid (which indicates irritation in the spinal canal); in the case of inflammation of the arachnoid membrane (the contrast medium may increase the severity of the inflammation); or when there is increased intracranial pressure (tapping of the subarachnoid space with needle insertion may cause complications as the pressure equalizes between areas of the brain and spinal cord).

Chapter 6: Image Acquisition and Evaluation

Selection of Technical Factors

1. In order to make a noticeable change in the density of an image, the mAs should be increased by a minimum of

    (A) 20%.
    (B) 30%.
    (C) 50%.
    (D) 100%.

2. Increasing kVp affects density by

    1. increasing the penetrability of the beam.
    2. increasing the production of scattered photons.
    3. increasing the number of photons produced.

    (A) 1 and 2 only
    (B) 1 and 3 only
    (C) 2 and 3 only
    (D) 1, 2, and 3

3. A patient presents in the emergency department after a fall. The physician orders a radiograph of the lumbar spine. The technique chart calls for a technique of 50 mAs, 75 kVp, and 40" SID. Due to other vital equipment in the room, an SID of 50" must be used. Which of the following mAs selections must be made in order to maintain radiographic density?

    (A) 32
    (B) 40
    (C) 63
    (D) 78

4. Increasing filtration will require an increase in what factor in order to maintain film density?

    (A) mAs
    (B) Distance
    (C) Grid ratio
    (D) Collimation

5. Tightly collimating to the area of interest can reduce the density seen on a finished film due to

    (A) a decrease in the amount of photoelectric absorption.
    (B) a decrease in the amount of scatter reaching the image receptor.
    (C) the absorption of off-focus radiation by the collimator.
    (D) an increase in the penetrating ability of the X-ray beam.

6. Assuming that the same technique is used to perform an AP lumbar spine exam on each of the following patients, which resulting film would demonstrate the greatest amount of density?

    (A) A bodybuilder measuring 21 cm
    (B) An obese child measuring 21 cm
    (C) A bodybuilder measuring 34 cm
    (D) An obese adult measuring 34 cm

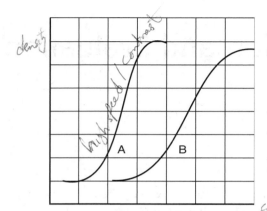

7. Which of the following statements is true about the D log E curve shown above?

    (A) Film A will require increased patient dose compared to Film B.

    (B) Film A will exhibit decreased contrast compared to Film B.

    (C) Film A will exhibit increased density compared to Film B.

    (D) Film A will exhibit decreased detail compared to Film B.

8. Which one of the following combinations will demonstrate the greatest variation in film density across the long axis of the film?

    (A) Short SID and small film size

    (B) Long SID and small film size

    (C) Short SID and large film size

    (D) Long SID and large film size

9. With all other factors remaining the same, which combination of film factors will result in the greatest film density?

    (A) Small crystal size and thin emulsion layer

    (B) Large crystal size and thin emulsion layer

    (C) Small crystal size and thick emulsion layer

    (D) Large crystal size and thick emulsion layer

10. A patient is brought to the emergency department with a broken forearm. The patient's forearm measures 10 cm prior to casting and 14 cm after a fiberglass cast is applied. If the patient returns for a follow-up exam a week later, how should a manual technique be adjusted in order to produce a quality radiograph?

    (A) Set a 10 cm technique without any additional variation

    (B) Set a 10 cm technique and add 10 kVp for the cast

    (C) Set a 14 cm technique without any additional variation

    (D) Set a 14 cm technique and add 10 kVp for the cast

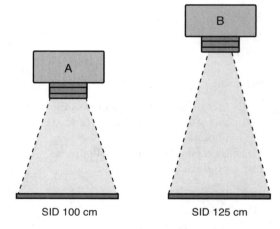

SID 100 cm   SID 125 cm

11. Referring to the tube-image receptor alignments illustrated above, which one of the following statements is true?

    (A) Alignment A would demonstrate increased recorded detail.

    (B) Alignment A would demonstrate an increased heel effect.

    (C) Alignment B would allow for a decrease in patient dose.

    (D) Alignment B would require an increased grid ratio.

GO ON TO THE NEXT PAGE

12. Which of the following adjustments will create a shorter scale of contrast?

    1. Increasing the focal spot size from small to large
    2. Increasing the OID from 4 cm to 10 cm
    3. Increasing beam restriction from 10 × 10 to 8 × 8

  (A) 1 and 2 only

  (B) 1 and 3 only

  (C) 2 and 3 only

  (D) 1, 2, and 3

13. Which of the following techniques would exhibit the shortest scale of contrast?

  (A) 50 mAs, 72 kVp, 10:1 grid, 40" SID, small focal spot

  (B) 63 mAs, 72 kVp, 12:1 grid, 40" SID, small focal spot

  (C) 117 mAs, 72 kVp, 16:1 grid, 50" SID, small focal spot

  (D) 50 mAs, 72 kVp, 8:1 grid, 35" SID, small focal spot

14. Which of the following changes will create many shades of gray across the finished image?

    1. Increasing kVp
    2. Decreasing grid ratio
    3. Increasing beam filtration

  (A) 1 and 2 only

  (B) 1 and 3 only

  (C) 2 and 3 only

  (D) 1, 2, and 3

15. Four identical AP lumbar spine radiographs are taken of four patients who have the four basic body types. The technique is adjusted to ensure a consistent density between all four images, and collimation is consistent between all four images. The radiograph of which body habitus would be most likely to demonstrate the longest scale of contrast?

  (A) Asthenic

  (B) Hyposthenic

  (C) Sthenic

  (D) Hypersthenic

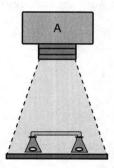 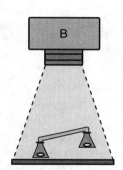

16. The tube, part, and image receptor arrangement demonstrated by B above would result in the anatomical structure appearing

  (A) normal sized.

  (B) elongated.

  (C) foreshortened.

  (D) minified.

GO ON TO THE NEXT PAGE

KAPLAN

17. A radiograph is produced at 25 mAs, 80 kVp, 40"
    SID, 1.2 mm focal spot, and using a 12:1 grid.
    Which of the following changes will increase
    recorded detail if the technique is adjusted to
    compensate for a change in exposure?

    1. Reduce focal spot size to 0.6 mm
    2. Increase grid ratio to 16:1
    3. Increase SID to 50"

    (A) 1 and 2 only
    (B) 1 and 3 only
    (C) 2 and 3 only
    (D) 1, 2, and 3

18. Which one of the following would be considered
    "involuntary" motion?

    (A) Peristalsis
    (B) Respiration
    (C) Blinking
    (D) Swallowing

19. Which of the following intensifying screen char-
    acteristics will result in the greatest recorded
    detail on a finished image?

    1. Decreased phosphor size
    2. Increased emulsion layer thickness
    3. Increased phosphor concentration

    (A) 1 and 2 only
    (B) 1 and 3 only
    (C) 2 and 3 only
    (D) 1, 2, and 3

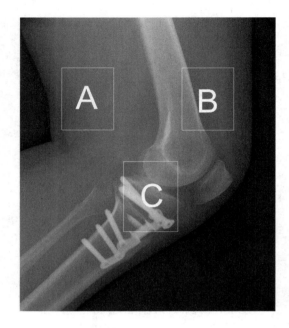

20. What would be the best choice for technical fac-
    tors if imaging the knee in the above image?

    (A) Use Chamber C with a +1 density adjustment
    (B) Use Chamber C with a -1 density adjustment
    (C) Use Chamber B without density adjustment
    (D) Measure and set a manual technique

21. A series of four exposures are taken of four objects
    using a 40" SID. Which object will appear largest
    on the finished film, given the original object size
    and OID listed?

    (A) 2" object; 4" OID
    (B) 2.5" object; 3" OID
    (C) 2.5" object; 8" OID
    (D) 3" object; 1" OID

GO ON TO THE NEXT PAGE

22. Which of the following would be the effects of moving from a 40" SID to a 48" SID?

    1. Decreased magnification
    2. Increased recorded detail
    3. Increased radiographic density

    (A) 1 and 2 only

    (B) 1 and 3 only

    (C) 2 and 3 only

    (D) 1, 2, and 3

23. A radiograph of an AP femur demonstrates fore-shortening of the bone. Which one of the following is the cause of this type of size misrepresentation?

    (A) Tube angle is too large

    (B) Tube angle is too short

    (C) Image receptor is not properly aligned to the central ray

    (D) Femur is not properly aligned to the central ray

24. Elongation occurs as a result of which of the following?

    1. The tube angle is greater than necessary.
    2. The image receptor is angled in relation to the central ray.
    3. The part being imaged is not properly aligned with the central ray.

    (A) 1 and 2 only

    (B) 1 and 3 only

    (C) 2 and 3 only

    (D) 1, 2, and 3

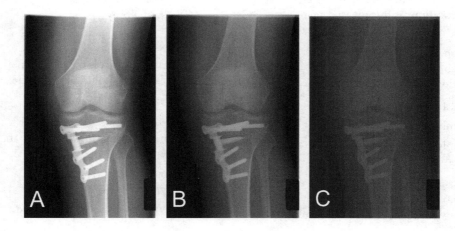

25. Which one of the three images above was taken with the greatest amount of filtration added to the X-ray beam?

    (A) A

    (B) B

    (C) C

    (D) All used the same filtration.

GO ON TO THE NEXT PAGE

26. Which of the following are major advantages of routinely using technique charts?

    1. Reduction in patient dose
    2. Reduction in repeat rate
    3. Consistent quality images

    (A) 1 and 2 only
    (B) 1 and 3 only
    (C) 2 and 3 only
    (D) 1, 2, and 3

27. What is the primary advantage of a variable kVp technique chart system compared to a fixed kVp technique chart system?

    (A) Decreased patient dose
    (B) Decreased tube wear
    (C) Increased image contrast
    (D) Increased image latitude

28. When setting a manual technique, a caliper is generally used to measure the body part. At which of the following locations is this measurement generally made?

    1. Through the thickest part
    2. Through the thinnest part
    3. Along the central ray

    (A) 1 and 2 only
    (B) 1 and 3 only
    (C) 2 and 3 only
    (D) 1, 2, and 3

29. Which factors must be manually set by the radiographer when utilizing an automatic exposure control technique?

    1. mA
    2. kVp
    3. Time

    (A) 1 and 2 only
    (B) 1 and 3 only
    (C) 2 and 3 only
    (D) 1, 2, and 3

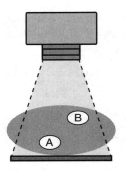

30. Which of the following statements would be true regarding the appearance of the finished image illustrated above?

    1. Object A would appear less magnified than Object B.
    2. Object A would display greater detail than Object B.
    3. Object A would receive greater exposure than Object B.

    (A) 1 and 2 only
    (B) 2 and 3 only
    (C) 1 and 3 only
    (D) 1, 2, and 3

31. The density controls on an automatic exposure control system should be used when

    (A) a correctly positioned exam produces a slightly underexposed image.
    (B) an exam is performed on a patient who has a hypersthenic body habitus.
    (C) an exam is performed on a patient who has a hyposthenic body habitus.
    (D) kVp is increased or decreased.

GO ON TO THE NEXT PAGE

32. The ionization chambers in a general radiographic room are adjusted so that a quality AP lumbar spine image is created when using automatic exposure control (AEC) and a collimated field size of 10" × 6". If the collimated field size is accidentally left open to a 14" × 17" field size, how would the image appear?

(A) Underexposed with better-than-expected contrast

(B) Underexposed with poorer-than-expected contrast

(C) Overexposed with better-than-expected contrast

(D) Overexposed with poorer-than-expected contrast

33. Which of the following pathologic conditions would require an increase in manual radiographic technique in order to maintain film density?

(A) Emphysema

(B) Pneumothorax

(C) Atelectasis

(D) Osteomalacia

34. What technical factor should be increased in order to compensate for the increased tissue density found in some pathologic conditions?

(A) kVp

(B) mA

(C) Time

(D) SID

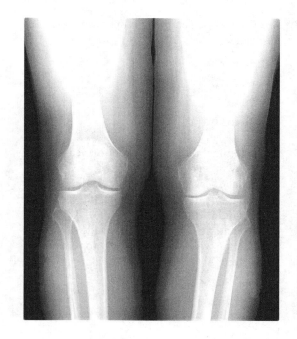

35.

The image above was obtained using automatic exposure control. Which of the following statements would explain the appearance of the above image?

(A) +1 density was selected.

(B) An incorrect detector was selected.

(C) Metallic artifacts altered exposure time.

(D) The patient moved during the exposure.

36. Which one of the following changes will increase the relative speed of an intensifying screen?

(A) Increase room temperature

(B) Increase SID

(C) Increase mAs

(D) Increase kVp

GO ON TO THE NEXT PAGE

KAPLAN

37. Relative film-screen speed is determined at what kVp range?

    (A) 50 to 60

    (B) 60 to 70

    (C) 70 to 80

    (D) 80 to 90

38. An abdominal radiograph is performed using the following technique: 40 mAs, 75 kVp, 48" SID, small focal spot, and a relative film-screen combination with a speed of 400. If a film-screen combination with a relative speed of 300 is utilized and no other change is made, what mAs setting will allow the density to remain unchanged?

    (A) 30

    (B) 46

    (C) 53

    (D) 80

39. Which of the following technical considerations are critical when using photostimulable imaging plates rather than film-screen combinations?

    1. Using the correct mAs
    2. Using the correct kVp
    3. Using the correct collimation

    (A) 1 and 2 only

    (B) 1 and 3 only

    (C) 2 and 3 only

    (D) 1, 2, and 3

A

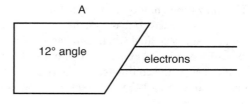

B

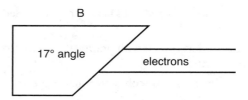

40. Which of the following statements are true regarding the anodes illustrated above?

    1. Anode A would lead to the patient receiving a smaller dose.
    2. Anode A would produce a smaller effective focal spot.
    3. Anode A would produce increased recorded detail.

    (A) 1 and 2 only

    (B) 1 and 3 only

    (C) 2 and 3 only

    (D) 1, 2, and 3

41. Use of an excessively low mAs setting when using digital radiography equipment will produce an image that displays

    (A) increased quantum mottle.

    (B) decreased density.

    (C) increased contrast.

    (D) increased detail.

GO ON TO THE NEXT PAGE

42. Sensitivity indicators for digital imaging systems such as S-number, EI, and LgM, are actually measurements of

    (A) density.

    (B) contrast.

    (C) detail.

    (D) exposure.

43. If 10 inches of each of the four types of tissues listed below were exposed to the same radiographic technique, which one would result in the greatest film density?

    (A) Lung

    (B) Fatty

    (C) Muscle

    (D) Bone

44. Which of the following pathological conditions would be considered a destructive pathology that requires a decrease in radiographic technique to compensate?

    (A) Ascites

    (B) Cirrhosis

    (C) Sclerosis

    (D) Pneumothorax

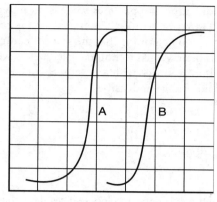

45. Which of the radiographic films exhibited above would require the highest radiographic technique setting in order to produce the same radiographic density?

    (A) A

    (B) B

    (C) Both films would require the same technical factors.

    (D) This information cannot be determined from this type of graph.

46. Although radiographic density can be adjusted by increasing and decreasing the SID, the main reason this technique is not used is that varying SID can also vary which of the following?

    1. Radiographic contrast
    2. Recorded detail
    3. Size distortion

    (A) 1 and 2 only

    (B) 1 and 3 only

    (C) 2 and 3 only

    (D) 1, 2, and 3

GO ON TO THE NEXT PAGE

KAPLAN)

47. A radiograph of a patient's ankle is produced at 10 mAs and 64 kVp. Upon viewing the radiograph, you determine that the scale of contrast is too high. Which technique listed below would result in an image with a lower scale of contrast and no change in density?

    (A) 10 mAs; 67 kVp
    (B) 5 mAs; 74 kVp
    (C) 20 mAs; 55 kVp
    (D) 10 mAs; 74 kVp

48. Which combination below will result in the greatest recorded detail on a finished image?

    (A) Long SID, long OID, large focal spot size
    (B) Long SID, short OID, large focal spot size
    (C) Long SID, short OID, small focal spot size
    (D) Short SID, short OID, small focal spot size

49. Which of the following alignments will result in the maximum reduction in the amount of distortion on a finished radiograph?

    (A) Part aligned parallel to image receptor and perpendicular to central ray
    (B) Part aligned perpendicular to image receptor and parallel to central ray
    (C) Part aligned perpendicular to image receptor and perpendicular to central ray
    (D) Part aligned parallel to image receptor and parallel to central ray

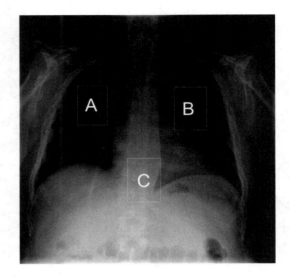

50. The radiograph above was performed using automatic exposure control (AEC); Detectors A and B were selected. If the examination is repeated using AEC, what change should be made prior to making the exposure?

    (A) Select Detectors A and C
    (B) Select Detector C only
    (C) Set the density control to +1
    (D) Set the density control to -1

51. If a green-sensitive film is accidentally used with a blue-emitting screen, the resulting image will be

    (A) white.
    (B) lighter than expected.
    (C) darker than expected.
    (D) black.

GO ON TO THE NEXT PAGE

52. Which of the following are effects of increased intensifying screen conversion efficiency?

    1. Increased noise
    2. Decreased technique requirements
    3. Decreased recorded detail

    (A) 1 and 2 only

    (B) 1 and 3 only

    (C) 2 and 3 only

    (D) 1, 2, and 3

53. As kVp increases, the percentage of which of the following types of X-ray interactions also increases?

    (A) Photoelectric

    (B) Compton

    (C) Coherent

    (D) Thompson

54. Radiographic technique must sometimes be increased when the X-ray beam is tightly collimated due to

    (A) a decrease in the amount of scatter reaching the image receptor.

    (B) the difficulty in penetrating the collimator shutters.

    (C) a decrease in the production of off-focus radiation.

    (D) a smaller effective focal spot size.

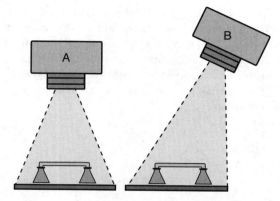

55. Which statement is true regarding the two tube alignments illustrated above?

    (A) Alignment A would result in increased recorded detail.

    (B) Alignment B would result in foreshortening.

    (C) Alignment A would result in foreshortening.

    (D) Alignment B would result in increased recorded detail.

56. Utilizing the air-gap technique will result in which of the following changes on the finished radiograph?

    1. Increased contrast
    2. Decreased detail
    3. Increased density

    (A) 1 and 2 only

    (B) 1 and 3 only

    (C) 2 and 3 only

    (D) 1, 2, and 3

GO ON TO THE NEXT PAGE

KAPLAN

57. A radiograph of an AP cervical spine is performed portably at 10 mAs and 70 kVp using an 8:1 grid. The cervical spine is imaged again in the general radiography department, this time using a 12:1 grid. What should be the mAs setting in order to compensate for the change in grid ratio?

(A) 6.5

(B) 8

(C) 12.5

(D) 15

58. Which of the following grid errors will result in a decrease in density along the right and left edges of the image?

1. Off focus
2. Off center
3. Upside down

(A) 1 and 2 only

(B) 1 and 3 only

(C) 2 and 3 only

(D) 1, 2, and 3

59. An AP pelvis radiograph is performed at 25 mAs and 75 kVp at a distance of 40". If the SID is increased to 60", what should be the mAs setting in order to compensate for the increased SID?

(A) 11

(B) 16

(C) 38

(D) 56

60. Why should the small focal spot be used only when highly detailed images are desired?

1. More X-rays can be produced with a small focal spot.
2. Exposure time must be reduced when using a small focal spot.
3. Heat is focused on a smaller area when using a small focal spot.

(A) 1 and 2 only

(B) 1 and 3 only

(C) 2 and 3 only

(D) 1, 2, and 3

61. An image is produced using a filter that totals 2.5 mm Al. If an additional 1.5 mm Al is added to the tube and radiographic technique is adjusted to compensate, how will the new images look when compared to the original images?

1. Decreased contrast
2. Increased noise
3. Decreased density

(A) 1 and 2 only

(B) 1 and 3 only

(C) 2 and 3 only

(D) 1, 2, and 3

62. An image of an AP thoracic spine is produced that displays a great deal of quantum mottle. Which of the changes listed below will reduce the appearance of quantum mottle?

1. Use of a higher mAs technique
2. Use of a lower kVp technique
3. Use of a slower speed image receptor

(A) 1 and 2 only

(B) 1 and 3 only

(C) 2 and 3 only

(D) 1, 2, and 3

GO ON TO THE NEXT PAGE

63. A radiograph of which anatomical structure listed below would demonstrate the greatest amount of distortion?

    (A) Hand
    (B) Knee
    (C) Pelvis
    (D) Ankle

64. To most effectively utilize the properties of the heel effect, toward what side of the patient should the cathode be positioned for an AP femur examination?

    (A) Superior
    (B) Inferior
    (C) On the patient's right side
    (D) On the patient's left side

65. The most common cause of motion blur on a radiograph is

    (A) tube movement.
    (B) image receptor movement.
    (C) patient motion.
    (D) grid oscillation.

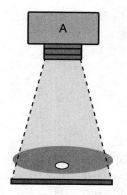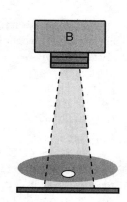

66. Which of the following statements is true regarding the two different X-ray beam arrangements shown above?

    (A) Arrangement B will result in increased density.
    (B) Arrangement B will result in increased contrast.
    (C) Arrangement B will result in increased detail.
    (D) Arrangement B will result in increased distortion.

67. What is the most important radiographic technique modification needed for pediatric radiography?

    (A) High kVp technique
    (B) High mAs technique
    (C) Short SID setting
    (D) Short time setting

68. The main reason intensifying screens are used in film-based radiography is to

    (A) increase recorded detail.
    (B) decrease patient dose.
    (C) protect radiographic film.
    (D) reduce kVp requirements.

GO ON TO THE NEXT PAGE ⟩

KAPLAN

69. A bone tumor located in the right shoulder will appear largest when the patient is placed in what position?

   (A) AP
   (B) PA
   (C) Right lateral
   (D) Left lateral

70. An AP pelvis exam is performed at 250 mA, 0.2 seconds, and 70 kVp. After reviewing the image, you determine that it is under-penetrated and needs to be repeated with an increased technique. Which of the techniques below would produce the desired density by following the 15 percent rule?

   (A) 288 mA, 0.2 seconds, 70 kVp
   (B) 250 mA, 0.23 seconds, 70 kVp
   (C) 250 mA, 0.2 seconds, 81 kVp
   (D) 325 mA, 0.2 seconds, 81 kVp

71. What is the primary advantage of using direct digital radiography over using photostimulable phosphor plates?

   (A) Nearly immediate results
   (B) Ability to adjust contrast electronically
   (C) Ability to adjust density electronically
   (D) Less expensive

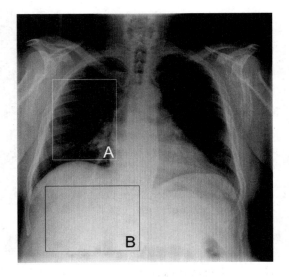

72. What is the primary reason that radiographic contrast is different in areas A and B shown above?

   (A) Use of different grids
   (B) kVp variations
   (C) Subject factors
   (D) Heel effect

73. Computed radiography systems that utilize photostimulable phosphor (PSP) imaging plates are designed to mimic the speed of a film/screen system in what range?

   (A) 50 to 100
   (B) 100 to 200
   (C) 200 to 400
   (D) 400 to 800

GO ON TO THE NEXT PAGE

74. When comparing film-screen and computed radiography systems, which of the following statements are true?

   1. Film/screen displays greater spatial resolution than computed radiography.
   2. Computed radiography displays greater contrast resolution than film-screen.
   3. Computed radiography results in less size distortion than film-screen.

   (A) 1 and 2 only
   (B) 1 and 3 only
   (C) 2 and 3 only
   (D) 1, 2, and 3

75. What is the most significant advantage of using solid-state detectors rather than photostimulable phosphor plates in digital radiography?

   (A) Collimation is not necessary.
   (B) Handling cassettes is not necessary.
   (C) Marking images is not necessary.
   (D) Centering the X-ray tube is not necessary.

76. An exposure is made at 40 mAs, 85 kVp, 45" SID, 8:1 grid, and small focal spot. If the grid ratio is increased to 12:1, which of the following changes will maintain radiographic density?

   (A) Increase the mAs to 55
   (B) Increase the kVp to 98
   (C) Increase the SID to 61"
   (D) Increase the focal spot size to "Large"

77. An AP pelvis radiograph is produced at 25 mAs, 85 kVp, 50" SID, and large focal spot size. If the image needs to be repeated in order to increase contrast, which one of the following techniques should be utilized to increase contrast while maintaining radiographic density?

   (A) 39 mAs, 85 kVp, 40" SID, large focal spot
   (B) 25 mAs, 98 kVp, 50" SID, small focal spot
   (C) 50 mAs, 72 kVp, 50" SID, small focal spot
   (D) 25 mAs, 72 kVp, 50" SID, large focal spot

78. An AP projection of the lumbar spine will display greater recorded detail than a PA projection due to

   (A) a reduction in scatter production.
   (B) a decreased OID.
   (C) the ability to reduce kVp.
   (D) the need for a higher grid ratio.

79. Quantum mottle can be corrected only by

   (A) increasing kVp.
   (B) increasing speed screen.
   (C) increasing mAs.
   (D) increasing SID.

80. An AP shoulder exam is performed at 200 mA, 0.1 seconds, and 72 kVp. Which one of the techniques listed below adheres to the reciprocity law?

   (A) 100 mA, 0.2 seconds, 72 kVp
   (B) 200 mA, 0.1 seconds, 83 kVp
   (C) 50 mA, 0.3 seconds, 72 kVp
   (D) 400 mA, 0.2 seconds, 61 kVp

GO ON TO THE NEXT PAGE

KAPLAN

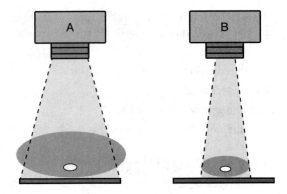

81. Which one of the following statements is true regarding the two patients being examined in the illustration above?

    (A) The image in Scenario A will display increased contrast.

    (B) The image in Scenario B will display increased recorded detail.

    (C) The image in Scenario A will display decreased magnification.

    (D) The image in Scenario B will display decreased latitude.

82. Film A is manufactured with a faster speed than Film B. If all other factors are equal, what change in technique will be required to change from Film A to Film B in order to maintain film density and contrast?

    (A) Increase kVp

    (B) Decrease kVp

    (C) Increase mAs

    (D) Decrease mAs

83. Most manufacturers of digital radiography systems recommend that a grid be used whenever a kVp is set above what level?

    (A) 70

    (B) 80

    (C) 90

    (D) 100

84. What is the minimum change in kVp necessary to produce a noticeable change in radiographic density?

    (A) 4%

    (B) 15%

    (C) 30%

    (D) 50%

85. Which type of radiographic technique chart would typically result in the highest patient dose?

    (A) Variable kilovoltage chart

    (B) Fixed kilovoltage chart

    (C) High kilovoltage chart

    (D) Automatic exposure chart

86. Decreasing the thickness of an anatomical structure through the use of a compression paddle or compression band will result in which of the following?

    1. Increased radiographic contrast
    2. Decreased recorded detail
    3. Decreased patient dose

    (A) 1 and 2 only

    (B) 1 and 3 only

    (C) 2 and 3 only

    (D) 1, 2, and 3

GO ON TO THE NEXT PAGE

A

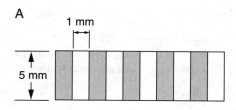

B

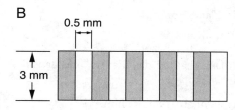

C

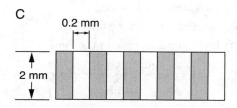

87. Which one of the grids illustrated above will most effectively improve radiographic contrast?

(A) A

(B) B

(C) C

(D) All grids pictured here are equal.

88. Which one of the following adjustments will reduce shape distortion?

(A) Place the central ray directly over the anatomy of interest.

(B) Move the anatomy of interest farther from the X-ray table.

(C) Angle the anatomy of interest 45° to the image receptor.

(D) Move the X-ray tube closer to the anatomy of interest.

89. The most critical factor to consider when using automatic exposure devices is

(A) setting the correct time.

(B) using the appropriate SID.

(C) correctly positioning the patient.

(D) setting the correct mAs.

90. What is the minimum kVp necessary to visualize the outline and lumen of a barium-filled colon?

(A) 69

(B) 74

(C) 90

(D) 104

GO ON TO THE NEXT PAGE

Image Processing and Quality Assurance

1. What is the optimal temperature at which radiographic film should be stored?

   (A) 55 to 68°F

   (B) 68 to 78°F

   (C) 78 to 88°F

   (D) Over 88°F

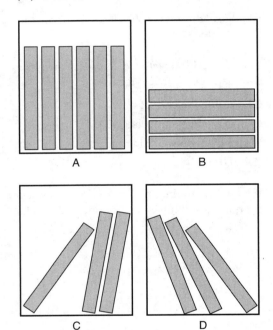

2. Which one of the configurations above is optimal for film storage?

   (A) A

   (B) B

   (C) C

   (D) D

3. Chemical fog is caused by which of the following?

   1. Increased water replenishment
   2. Increased development temperature
   3. Increased chemical concentration

   (A) 1 and 2 only

   (B) 1 and 3 only

   (C) 2 and 3 only

   (D) 1, 2, and 3

4. Artifacts that are classified as "plus densities" appear as

   (A) light areas on the film.

   (B) dark areas on the film.

   (C) detailed areas on the film.

   (D) high-contrast areas on the film.

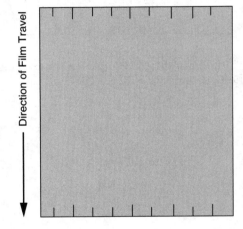

5. The most likely cause of the marks along the leading and trailing edge of a film as illustrated by the image above is

   (A) guide shoes.

   (B) dryer rollers.

   (C) entrance rollers.

   (D) developer rollers.

GO ON TO THE NEXT PAGE

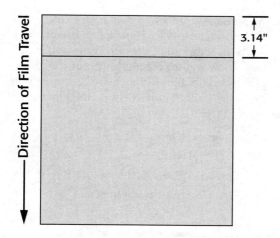

6. The cause of the artifact shown above is

   (A) improperly positioned crossover racks.
   (B) dirt buildup on rollers.
   (C) dryer temperature set too high.
   (D) incorrect placement of entrance roller.

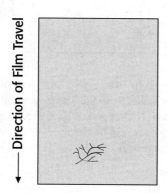

7. The cause of the artifact shown above is

   (A) dirt in the cassette.
   (B) water in the cassette.
   (C) static discharge.
   (D) chemical runoff.

8. Which of the following are acceptable methods of routinely placing patient identification on a radiographic image?

   1. Lead markers used during exposure
   2. Light exposure after exposure
   3. Permanent marker

   (A) 1 and 2 only
   (B) 1 and 3 only
   (C) 2 and 3 only
   (D) 1, 2, and 3

9. The latent image becomes visible for the first time in which part of the automatic processor?

   (A) Fixer
   (B) Wash
   (C) Developer
   (D) Dryer

10. What can happen if the temperature of the water in the wash tank is more than 5°F cooler than the temperature in the developer and fixer?

    (A) The film emulsion can crack.
    (B) The film may feel "sticky."
    (C) The film may have a "milky" appearance.
    (D) The film base may become soft.

11. Undeveloped silver halide crystals are removed from radiographic film in which part of the automatic film processor?

    (A) Fixer
    (B) Dryer
    (C) Developer
    (D) Wash

GO ON TO THE NEXT PAGE

KAPLAN

12. If the wash tank of the automatic processor does not adequately do its job, how will the film appear after several years?

(A) Milky white

(B) Yellow

(C) Black

(D) Clear

13. The dryer in an automatic processor is primarily responsible for which of the following?

   1. Removing undeveloped silver halide crystals
   2. Sealing the supercoat
   3. Hardening the emulsion

(A) 1 and 2 only

(B) 1 and 3 only

(C) 2 and 3 only

(D) 1, 2, and 3

14. Which part of the automatic film processor controls the amount of time the film spends in each chemical solution?

(A) Replenishment system

(B) Recirculation system

(C) Transportation system

(D) Silver recovery system

15. Whenever an automatic processor is cleaned and new developer chemicals are poured into the developer tank, the chemicals are much too active to begin developing films immediately. What should be done first to "season" the processor chemicals before attempting to develop patient images?

(A) Run 25 to 30 unexposed films through the processor

(B) Wait a minimum of 6 hours before running films

(C) Add a "starter" solution to the replenishment solution

(D) Add approximately 2 liters of the old developer chemicals to the tank

16. An automatic processor is set up for volume replenishment and lengthwise film orientation (with the long end of the film against the feed tray). How will the replenishment of chemicals be affected if a film is run crosswise through the processor (with the short end of the film against the feed tray)?

(A) Under-replenishment

(B) Over-replenishment

(C) Correct replenishment

(D) Film placement is unimportant.

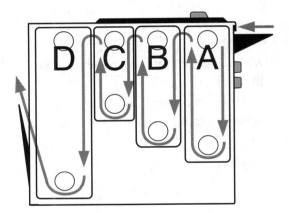

17. If chemicals from a certain tank get into one of the other tanks in an automatic processor, processing is severely changed. Which chemical exchange listed below would be the most devastating to an automatic processor?

(A) C to A

(B) A to B

(C) B to C

(D) B to A

GO ON TO THE NEXT PAGE ▷

18. Which of the following are tasks performed by the circulation system of an automatic processor?

    1. Chemical replenishment
    2. Chemical mixing
    3. Temperature maintenance

    (A) 1 and 2 only
    (B) 1 and 3 only
    (C) 2 and 3 only
    (D) 1, 2, and 3

19. After a film is inserted into an automatic processor, how does the transport system notify the radiographer that it is safe to either turn on a light or add another film to the processor?

    (A) A "ready light" is illuminated.
    (B) An audible noise is made.
    (C) An entrance roller begins to turn.
    (D) A transport "gate" is lowered.

20. Which type of replenishment should be used in a small medical office that does not produce a large quantity of films during the day?

    (A) Volume
    (B) Standard
    (C) Flood
    (D) Extended

21. In order to prevent dust and dirt from collecting inside a cassette during film loading, the cassette should

    (A) be cleaned after every use.
    (B) be examined with a black light after every use.
    (C) never be touched with bare hands.
    (D) never be opened completely.

22. Which of the following changes to the development chemistry of an automatic processor will cause an increase in radiographic density on a processed image?

    1. Increased development time
    2. Increased developer temperature
    3. Increased developer concentration

    (A) 1 and 2 only
    (B) 1 and 3 only
    (C) 2 and 3 only
    (D) 1, 2, and 3

23. Which one of the following automatic processor components is NOT used with a daylight processing system?

    (A) Feed tray
    (B) Dryer
    (C) Crossover assembly
    (D) Temperature regulator

24. All radiographic images MUST be marked with which one of the following?

    (A) Patient's age
    (B) Radiographer's name
    (C) Patient's date of birth
    (D) "Right" or "Left" identification

25. This part of the processor should be removed and cleaned daily before the first images of the day are developed.

    (A) Feed tray
    (B) Crossover assembly
    (C) Dryer rollers
    (D) Processor lid

GO ON TO THE NEXT PAGE

26. When an automatic processor is shut down at the end of the day,

    (A) the developer tank should be completely drained.
    (B) the fixer tank should be completely drained.
    (C) the processor lid should be raised.
    (D) the developer filter should be replaced.

27. The mid-density point on a processor control chart should not vary by more than

    (A) ± 0.05.
    (B) ± 0.10.
    (C) ± 0.15.
    (D) ± 0.20.

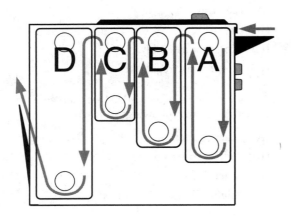

28. In which one of the following sections of the automatic processor would the film be subjected to the greatest amount of heat?

    (A) A
    (B) B
    (C) C
    (D) D

29. In sensitometry, what is the name for the measurement of the unexposed, clear area of the film?

    (A) Density difference
    (B) Dmax
    (C) Base + Fog
    (D) Dmin

30. Which two sections of an automatic processor are primarily responsible for the archiving quality of a film?

    (A) Developer and fixer
    (B) Wash and dryer
    (C) Fixer and wash
    (D) Developer and dryer

31. The majority of monitors used to view digital images are able to provide resolution in what range?

    (A) 1 to 2 lp/mm
    (B) 4 to 6 lp/mm
    (C) 8 to 12 lp/mm
    (D) 15 to 20 lp/mm

32. Which one of the following combinations will provide the best digital image resolution?

    (A) Large pixel size and large matrix size
    (B) Large pixel size and small matrix size
    (C) Small pixel size and small matrix size
    (D) Small pixel size and large matrix size

33. When the digital image has been processed and the image appears on a monitor, the contrast can be modified electronically. Which statement below correctly describes the digital contrast control?

    (A) Increased window width increases contrast
    (B) Increased window width decreases contrast
    (C) Decreased window levels increase contrast
    (D) Decreased window levels decrease density

GO ON TO THE NEXT PAGE

34. Which of the following are benefits of utilizing a PACS for digital image storage?

    1. Redundant storage
    2. Access from multiple locations
    3. Decreased time for image retrieval

    (A) 1 and 2 only
    (B) 1 and 3 only
    (C) 2 and 3 only
    (D) 1, 2, and 3

35. An essential part of a PACS is the ability of different pieces of equipment from different vendors to communicate with each other. What is the name of the common "language" used by digital imaging equipment?

    (A) SMPTE
    (B) DICOM
    (C) NEMA
    (D) RIS

36. What percentage of the latent image will be lost if a photostimulable phosphor plate is not processed within 8 hours of exposure?

    (A) 0%
    (B) 25%
    (C) 50%
    (D) 100%

Criteria for Image Evaluation

1. An image is produced that lacks sufficient radiographic density. What should be adjusted in order to produce an optimal radiograph?

    (A) mAs should be increased by a factor of 2.
    (B) mAs should be decreased by a factor of 2.
    (C) kVp should be increased by a factor of 2.
    (D) kVp should be decreased by a factor of 2.

2. The primary effect that the use of a grid has on the quality of the completed image is

    (A) increased density.
    (B) increased detail.
    (C) increased contrast.
    (D) decreased motion.

3. A radiograph of a lateral cervical spine is produced portably using a film-screen technique and hung on a view box for evaluation. Upon inspection, an area of unsharpness is observed in only one small section of the image. The most probable cause of this abnormality is

    (A) an increased OID due to the distance of the cervical spine from the film.
    (B) poor film-screen contact due to an old or damaged screen.
    (C) excessive patient motion due to poor patient communication.
    (D) a decrease in SID due to a portable technique.

4. An abdominal radiograph is produced on a patient in the morning and again on the same patient in the afternoon. In the morning the technologist performs an AP projection of the patient's abdomen and in the afternoon the technologist performs a PA radiograph. Which one of the following statements would describe the visual difference between the two images?

    (A) The AP projection will demonstrate increased contrast in the stomach.
    (B) The AP projection will demonstrate increased density of the liver.
    (C) The PA projection will demonstrate increased size distortion of the kidneys.
    (D) The PA projection will demonstrate increased detail of the spine.

GO ON TO THE NEXT PAGE

5. Directing the central ray directly on the anatomy of interest in a perpendicular orientation will reduce which types of distortion on a completed image?

   1. Magnification
   2. Elongation
   3. Foreshortening

   (A) 1 and 2 only
   (B) 1 and 3 only
   (C) 2 and 3 only
   (D) 1, 2, and 3

6. Every radiographic image should include which type of anatomical marker?

   (A) Superior or Inferior
   (B) Right or Left
   (C) AP or PA
   (D) Upright or Recumbent

7. Blurring of the radiographic image across the entire film would most likely be the result of

   (A) involuntary muscle movement.
   (B) voluntary muscle movement.
   (C) poor film-screen contact.
   (D) an image processing malfunction.

8. Hundreds of faint, very thin lines running parallel to each other are seen on a completed radiograph. The cause of these artifacts is

   (A) grid lines.
   (B) processor rollers.
   (C) crossover racks.
   (D) static discharge.

9. Which one of the following malfunctions will cause fog on a complete image?

   (A) Decreased processor temperature
   (B) Inadequate developer replenishment
   (C) Dust inside a cassette
   (D) Cracks in the safelight filter

10. How does noise appear on a radiograph?

    (A) An image with increased density
    (B) An image with decreased density
    (C) An image with a grainy appearance
    (D) An image with a blurry appearance

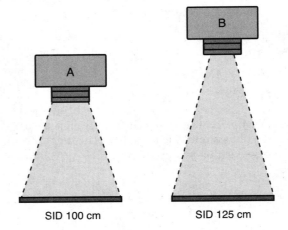

SID 100 cm   SID 125 cm

11. Which of the following statements is true regarding the two configurations shown above if all other factors remain unchanged?

    (A) Arrangement A will result in greater detail on a finished image.
    (B) Arrangement A will result in greater density on a finished image.
    (C) Arrangement B will result in greater patient dose.
    (D) Arrangement B will result in greater motion blur.

GO ON TO THE NEXT PAGE

12. A radiographic image of an elbow is performed on a patient who fell from a skateboard. Upon reviewing the image, the radiologist asks for an additional film with increased contrast. Which change listed below will fill the radiologist's need?

    (A) Increase kVp and lower mAs

    (B) Decrease kVp and increase mAs

    (C) Increase SID and increase mAs

    (D) Decrease SID and decrease mAs

13. A radiographic image of a pediatric chest is performed in the emergency department. Upon reviewing the image, a considerable amount of motion is detected and it is determined that the image will need to be repeated. If time is reduced to decrease the amount of motion seen on the completed image, which change below will compensate for the reduced time without making any other change to the image?

    (A) Increase kVp

    (B) Decrease SID

    (C) Utilize a faster speed screen

    (D) Increase mA

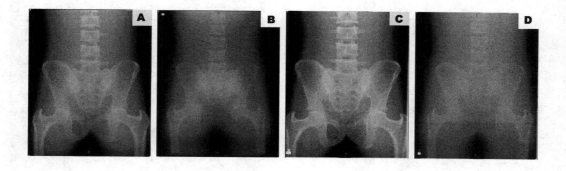

14. All of the images displayed above were produced with the same SID; which one was produced with the largest OID?

    (A) A

    (B) B

    (C) C

    (D) D

GO ON TO THE NEXT PAGE ⟩

KAPLAN)

15. While performing an AP axial projection of a clavicle, the technologist angles the X-ray tube 25° cephalic. How will this image appear when compared to an AP projection of the clavicle?

    1. Increased distortion
    2. Decreased superimposition
    3. Decreased magnification

    (A) 1 and 2 only
    (B) 1 and 3 only
    (C) 2 and 3 only
    (D) 1, 2, and 3

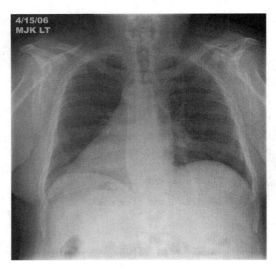

16. Which one of the following types of identification is missing on the image displayed above?

    (A) Exam date
    (B) Patient identifier
    (C) Anatomical side indicator
    (D) Technologist identifier

17. A lateral skull projection is performed on a patient with Paget disease using a manually set radiographic technique. If the technologist overlooks the Paget disease indication on the exam order and sets a normal technique, how will the image appear?

    (A) More elongated than expected
    (B) More dense than expected
    (C) Less dense than expected
    (D) Less noisy than expected

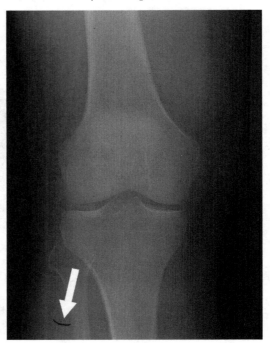

18. The cause of the artifact identified by the white arrow is

    (A) rough handling.
    (B) static discharge.
    (C) pressure prior to exposure.
    (D) pressure after exposure.

GO ON TO THE NEXT PAGE

19. Film that is used after its expiration date will display which of the following?

    1. Increased fog
    2. Decreased contrast
    3. Decreased density

    (A) 1 and 2 only

    (B) 1 and 3 only

    (C) 2 and 3 only

    (D) 1, 2, and 3

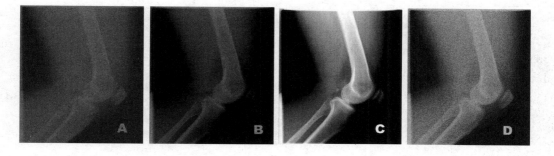

20. Which one of the images displayed above demonstrates the greatest amount of noise?

    (A) A

    (B) B

    (C) C

    (D) D

21. What are the benefits of using a 10' SID for a chest radiograph rather than a 6' SID?

    1. Increased detail
    2. Decreased magnification
    3. Decreased mAs requirements

    (A) 1 and 2 only

    (B) 1 and 3 only

    (C) 2 and 3 only

    (D) 1, 2, and 3

22. Storing X-ray film in an exam room can result in increased density due to

    (A) chemical fog.

    (B) radiation fog.

    (C) temperature fog.

    (D) safelight fog.

GO ON TO THE NEXT PAGE

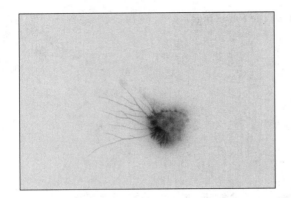

24. Which one of the following pathological conditions will require a reduction in technique in order to maintain radiographic density?

    (A) Osteoporosis

    (B) Aortic aneurysm

    (C) Ascites

    (D) Pleural effusion

23. The cause of the artifact displayed above is

    (A) pressure.

    (B) dirt in the cassette.

    (C) poor film/screen contact.

    (D) static.

Answers and Explanations

Selection of Technical Factors

1. The correct answer is (B).

It is difficult for the human eye to make out a density difference on a radiograph if the change in density is less than 30 percent. A change of 50 percent in mAs would be more likely to demonstrate a change in density, but it would not be the minimum change needed. Doubling the mAs by increasing it 100 percent is the preferred method of making changes in radiographic density, but once again it is not the *minimum* requirement to see an observable change.

2. The correct answer is (A).

Increasing kVp will increase the average energy of the X-ray photons being produced but does not affect the *number* of photons created in the anode. mAs is the primary factor that controls the number of X-ray photons that are produced. Increasing the kVp also increases the likelihood of a scatter interaction inside the patient's body. This leads to an increase in the amount of scatter reaching the image receptor and will increase the density of the image.

3. The correct answer is (D).

The exposure maintenance formula (also known as the direct square law) must be used to solve this problem (New mAs = Old mAs × New Distance^2/Old Distance^2). Rooted in the inverse square law, this formula follows the general rule that radiation intensity decreases as distance increases. However, instead of stating a change in radiation intensity, the exposure maintenance formula describes the change in mAs necessary to compensate for the change in distance. The exposure maintenance formula does not describe an inverse relationship; in other words, if distance increases, the mAs will also need to increase in order to compensate.

4. The correct answer is (A).

Adding anything to the useful beam attenuates the beam and will require an increase in technique to compensate; mAs is the factor of choice to use when increasing technique. Increasing the filtration attenuates the beam just like an increase in grid ratio, table thickness, or patient thickness would.

5. The correct answer is (B).

Restricting the X-ray beam reduces the area where scattered radiation is produced. A reduction in scattered radiation reaching the film results in a corresponding reduction in film density. The amount of scatter that reaches the image receptor is the critical component to fluctuations of density caused by collimation. Since the useful beam does not travel through the collimator shutters, the collimator is an influencing factor only on the area being exposed, the amount of scatter production, and ultimately the amount of scatter reaching the finished film. The collimator is not a *direct* cause of density increase or decrease.

6. The correct answer is (B).

Because the technique remains constant for all four individuals, the important factor used to determine density is the amount of radiation that reaches the image receptor. The type and volume of tissue being exposed determine how much of the beam will be absorbed prior to reaching the film. The patients who measure 21 cm will be easier to penetrate, and fat is easier to penetrate than muscle. Therefore, the patient who measures 21 cm with a greater amount of fatty tissue will be easiest to penetrate and will result in the film with the greatest density.

7. The correct answer is (C).

Film A is faster than Film B and exhibits increased contrast. The horizontal axis on this D log E curve represents exposure, while the vertical axis represents density. As exposure increases (from left to right), density increases (from bottom to top). Therefore, it takes less exposure to Film A to see a visible change in density and patient dose can be decreased.

8. The correct answer is (C).

The anode heel effect refers to the variation of radiation intensity from one side of the X-ray tube to the other. Radiation intensity and resulting film density are greater on the cathode side of the tube as compared to the anode side. Two factors under the control of radiographers can affect the severity of the anode heel effect: SID and film size. The shorter the SID and the larger the film size, the greater the anode heel effect becomes. A good rule of thumb is to think about how open the collimators are in a certain situation; the more widely open the collimators are, the greater the anode heel effect will be. The combination of a short SID and a large film size require that the collimators be open wider than any other combination listed.

9. The correct answer is (D).

As silver halide crystal size increases, the likelihood of an interaction with an X-ray photon increases. In the same way, if the emulsion layer (which contains the silver halide crystals) is increased in thickness, there is a greater chance of photon interaction. If more photons interact with a greater number of silver halide crystals, more darkening will occur and density will increase.

10. The correct answer is (C).

The cast should be treated as an extension of the patient's anatomy. It should be measured and a technique set based on the thickness of the cast. There is no need to make any other changes based on the addition of the cast, regardless of material. The only possible exception is for a wet plaster cast, which may require an increase in technique.

11. The correct answer is (B).

A shorter SID requires that the collimator be opened wider to cover the entire image receptor. As the collimator is opened, the effects of the heel effect become more evident. Increased SID leads to increased detail but will require an increase in technique to compensate for the increased distance.

12. The correct answer is (C).

Contrast is degraded when scattered radiation strikes the image receptor and adds a cloudy density to the finished image. Increasing the OID will cause scattered radiation to miss the image receptor and therefore improve the contrast. This is called the *"air-gap technique."* Tightly collimating reduces the production of scattered radiation inside the patient's body and thus reduces the amount of scattered radiation that strikes the image receptor. Focal spot sizes do not significantly affect radiographic contrast.

13. The correct answer is (C).

The two controlling factors for contrast listed in this question are kVp and grid ratio. Because kVp is constant for all techniques, the one with the highest grid ratio would demonstrate the greatest contrast.

14. The correct answer is (D).

All of the changes listed will create many shades of gray across a finished image—in other words, will decrease the contrast. Increasing kVp increases the amount of scatter produced, decreasing the grid ratio inhibits the grid's ability to absorb scattered radiation, and increasing the amount of filtration increases the average energy of the X-ray beam, effectively increasing the average kVp coming from the tube.

15. The correct answer is (D).

The patient's body size is a determining factor in the amount of contrast seen on a finished image. A larger patient has a larger volume of tissue in which scatter radiation can be created, thus decreasing the contrast on the finished radiograph. Of the four basic body types, the largest and most likely to produce scattered radiation is the hypersthenic body habitus.

16. The correct answer is (C).

Foreshortening occurs whenever the anatomical structure is positioned at an angle to the image receptor and tube. In order for the anatomy to appear elongated, the tube must be angled in relation to the image receptor. Minification occurs in fluoroscopy, not general radiography.

17. The correct answer is (B).

The recorded detail can be improved by reducing the size of the focal spot, increasing the SID, or both. The focal spot is the area on the anode where X-rays are actually produced. The smaller this area is, the sharper the edges of objects will appear; this is a part of the "line focus principle." The angle of the anode can also affect the size of the focal spot as it exits the tube (also called the effective focal spot). The smaller the angle, the smaller the effective focal spot will be and the greater the recorded detail will appear. Increasing SID helps to improve recorded detail by minimizing the unsharpness around the edges of objects. You can demonstrate this for yourself by placing your hand in front of an overhead projector or other light source so that a shadow is cast on the wall. You will notice that as you move the light source away from the wall (increasing SID), the edges of your hand become more distinct. Grids do not affect recorded detail.

18. The correct answer is (A).

Involuntary motion is motion that cannot be controlled by the patient for even a short exposure time. Although it may be difficult, patients should be able to stop breathing, blinking, or swallowing for a short time. It would be impossible to ask a patient to stop the digestive system from working for even a short exposure.

19. The correct answer is (B).

Intensifying screens affect the recorded detail on the finished film through the effects of three characteristics. As phosphor size decreases, recorded detail increases; as the emulsion layer thickness decreases, recorded detail increases; and as the phosphors become more densely packed in the emulsion layer, recorded detail increases.

20. The correct answer is (D).

Due to the metal screws and plates in the patient's leg, automatic exposure control (AEC) would not be a good choice. Choice (C) would result in an underexposed image due to the fact that the majority of the chamber lies beneath soft tissue. The presence of metal would cause the AEC to continue the production of X-rays beyond what is needed and the image would be overexposed. Making a -1 density adjustment may lighten the film a bit, but setting a manual technique will ensure that a proper exposure is generated. This is one reason why taking a patient history prior to examining the patient is vitally important.

21. The correct answer is (C).

The first step in solving this problem is to determine the *magnification factor* for each exposure. The magnification factor (MF) is determined by using the formula MF = SID/SOD. The magnification factor is then multiplied by the original size of the object. For example, in exposure (A), MF = 40/36 and the resulting MF = 1.11. MF (1.11) is then multiplied by the original size of the object (2") to give a final answer of 2.22". If this same procedure is used for each of the four exposures, exposure (C) will provide the largest object size on the finished film, 3.13".

22. The correct answer is (A).

SID is a main controlling factor of magnification and detail. As SID increases, magnification decreases and detail increases. Using a large SID will not only improve recorded detail, but the smaller resulting magnification will allow large objects, such as wide lungs on a chest radiograph, to fit on one image receptor. Increasing SID with no compensation will reduce density; increasing SID with compensation will only maintain density.

23. The correct answer is (D).

Foreshortening is the misrepresentation of an object so that it appears shorter or smaller than it really is. This can occur only when the part is angled in relation to the central ray.

24. The correct answer is (A).

Elongation occurs whenever the central ray and image receptor are not properly aligned. This can occur when the tube is angled in relation to the image receptor or the image receptor is angled in relation to the central ray. If the part is not properly aligned to the central ray, the part will appear shorter than expected, or *"foreshortened."*

25. The correct answer is (C).

Increasing tube filtration increases the average kVp and increases the production of scatter. Increased scatter results in lower overall contrast. Image C displays the lowest contrast of the three images presented; therefore, it must be the image with the greatest amount of added filtration.

26. The correct answer is (D).

Technique charts should be used for all exposures, whether manual techniques are set or AEC is utilized. The use of a technique chart ensures that the highest quality image is produced using the lowest exposure. Proper use of a technique chart will ensure that image quality is consistent in density, detail, and contrast.

27. The correct answer is (C).

When using a variable kVp technique chart system, the radiographer is able to make very small adjustments to kVp that will improve the overall contrast of an image. When the kVp is "fixed" at a certain setting and mAs is adjusted to compensate for part thickness, the kVp is generally set to a higher setting that will produce more scattered radiation and degrade the contrast on the image. Decreased contrast is also referred to as increased latitude (D).

28. The correct answer is (B).

When making a measurement, the anatomy of interest must be measured so that an appropriate technique can be selected. The measurement is usually made by measuring along the path of the central ray as it enters and exits the patient. Another valid way of measuring is to measure the thickest part of the anatomy of interest to ensure that all anatomy is penetrated. Measuring the thinnest part may lead to underpenetration, decreased density, and a need to repeat the image.

29. The correct answer is (A).

The only factor controlled by automatic exposure control is time; the radiographer must still select the appropriate kVp and mA station. The AEC system will terminate an exposure when enough radiation has reached the image receptor to create an appropriate density on the film; it will keep the exposure running (increase the time) until this has occurred.

30. The correct answer is (A).

Object A is closer to the image receptor than object B. When the object-to-image receptor distance (OID) is decreased, magnification is decreased and recorded detail is increased.

31. The correct answer is (A).

Density controls (-3, -2, -1, 0, +1, +2, +3) should be used only to compensate for unexpected underexposure or overexposure due to patient pathology, anatomy, or positioning irregularities. AEC can automatically adjust for changes in patient thickness, body habitus, or changes in kVp, so it is unnecessary for the radiologist to set the density controls to shut off sooner or stay on longer.

32. The correct answer is (B).

Opening the collimators wider than necessary when using AEC will cause an increase in the amount of scatter production and a corresponding decrease in contrast on the completed image. The increase in scatter production will also cause the ionization chamber to sense an increase in the amount of radiation reaching the image receptor and the exposure will be terminated prematurely, thus causing an underexposed image.

33. The correct answer is (C).

Atelectasis, or "collapsed lung," is a condition in which a part of the chest cavity normally occupied by an air-filled lung is replaced by fluid or tissue. This increases the tissue density, making it more difficult to penetrate, and an increase in technique is needed to maintain film density. The other conditions listed result in a decrease in tissue density and would require a reduction in radiographic technique in order to maintain film density.

34. The correct answer is (A).

The problem associated with increased tissue density is a problem of penetration. Pathologic conditions such as *Paget disease* increase the density of the tissues and attenuate the X-ray beam to a greater extent than expected. kVp controls the penetrating power of the X-ray beam, so this factor should be increased in order to ensure that the beam is able to reach the image receptor.

35. The correct answer is (B).

For this exam, the center detector was selected (between the knees) and the exposure time was greatly reduced. AEC detectors are designed to terminate an exposure when a set amount of radiation has reached the image receptor. Since the X-ray beam was not adequately attenuated in the area of the selected detector, radiation easily reached it and the exposure was terminated prematurely.

36. The correct answer is (D).

Increasing kVp increases the likelihood that an incident X-ray photon will interact with the *phosphors* of the *intensifying screen*. This results in a more efficient screen, and therefore, a greater speed. No other factor under the control of the radiographer will affect the efficiency of the screen, although using screens in warm weather conditions (greater than 38°C) will result in less efficient X-ray/phosphor interactions and a slower overall screen.

37. The correct answer is (C).

Since kVp affects the efficiency of the film-screen combination, a range of kVp is selected by manufacturers when determining the relative speed of a film-screen system. Above and below this range the film-screen combination will respond differently, although this change will not be immediately apparent in the diagnostic range of kVp.

38. The correct answer is (C).

In order to determine the new mAs when a new screen is selected, the following formula is utilized:

$$= \frac{mAs_1}{mAs_2} \quad \frac{\text{Relative Speed}_2}{\text{Relative Speed}_1}$$

When the known quantities are substituted in the above formula it should look like this:

$$= \frac{40}{mAs_2} \quad \frac{300}{400}$$

Now multiply the original mAs by the original speed ($40 \times 400 = 16{,}000$) and divide by the new speed to determine the new mAs ($16{,}000/300 = 53$).

39. The correct answer is (C).

Photostimulable imaging plates are capable of compensating for relatively large variations in mAs, however, these plates are very sensitive to scattered radiation. Keeping the kVp set to an appropriate level and collimating to reduce the production of scatter will ensure that the best possible image is created.

40. The correct answer is (C).

A smaller anode angle will lead to a smaller effective focal spot size and increased recorded detail. In this case, Anode A has a 12° angle and Anode B has a 17° angle; therefore, Anode A will produce the smallest effective focal spot size and the greatest detail. The focal spot size does not have a noticeable effect on radiographic dose.

41. The correct answer is (A).

Quantum mottle is the grainy appearance displayed on images that lack a sufficient number of X-ray interactions. Because mAs primarily controls the number of X-ray photons that reach the image receptor, a lack of photons results in a lack of information on the finished image. The computer algorithms will attempt to compensate for the decrease on photons and boost the "density" of the image so the image will not appear to be underexposed.

42. The correct answer is (D).

Since digital imaging systems are able to manipulate the digital data in order to lighten or darken the finished image, the use of the term "density" to describe how much radiation has reached the image receptor is misleading. In digital imaging, the best way to determine if the correct technical factors have been used is to determine how much radiation has reached the image receptor. Different manufacturers use different terminology to describe the amount of radiation exposure to the image receptor, but most agree that an exposure of 1 mR is an appropriate level of radiation exposure needed to create a quality image.

43. The correct answer is (A).

Lung tissue, which contains air-filled sacs, would be the easiest for an X-ray to penetrate. Therefore, the amount of X-rays that would penetrate lung tissue and create a density on the finished film would be greater than the other tissues and would create the greatest density of any of the tissues listed. The tissues in answer choices (A) through (D) are listed in order of opacity—that is, from easiest to penetrate (lung) to most difficult (bone). When measuring and using a manual technique, it is important for radiographers to consider the patient's body habitus, including the predominant tissue in the patient's body. A muscular patient and an obese patient that measure the same thickness would not necessarily require the same technical factors.

44. The correct answer is (D).

A *pneumothorax* is characterized by free air in the chest cavity that pushes lung tissue out of the way. Since air is very easy to penetrate, the radiographic technique must be decreased in order to maintain an appropriate density. The other pathologies listed in this question are considered "*constructive*" pathologies because they require an increase in technique in order to compensate for an increase in tissue density.

45. The correct answer is (B).

A D log E curve like the one shown here is a graphical representation of how radiographic density and contrast are affected by changes in exposure (technical settings). In this case, the D log E curve shows that Film B would require an increase in exposure (horizontal line) to produce a desired radiographic density (vertical line).

46. The correct answer is (C).

The SID has no effect on contrast, however, it does affect the geometric factors of detail and distortion. Detail decreases and magnification (size distortion) increases as SID decreases. Because varying the SID to adjust the radiographic density of an image will also affect the appearance of anatomical structures on a finished radiograph, it would be a poor choice to use; using mAs to increase or decrease density is a far better choice.

47. The correct answer is (B).

Although answers (A), (B), and (D) would all result in a lower scale of contrast, only answer (B) adjusts mAs to compensate for the increase in kVp. Increasing the kVp by 15 percent effectively doubles the radiographic density as well as lowers the scale of contrast. Cutting the mAs in half also cuts the radiographic density in half without directly affecting image contrast. The net effect of these two changes is that the increase in kVp and the decrease in mAs cancel each other out, whereas the increase in kVp lowers the overall contrast of the image.

48. The correct answer is (C).

The combination of a long SID, short OID, and small focal spot size will result in the best possible recorded detail. Long SID and short OID ensure that the lowest possible magnification occurs, and a small focal spot results in less blurring of the edges of objects than would occur with a large focal spot.

49. The correct answer is (A).

When the anatomical part of interest is aligned perpendicular to the central ray and parallel to the image receptor, the only distortion that occurs is size distortion due to magnification. If the central ray is perpendicular to the image receptor and the anatomical part is positioned at an angle to either the central ray or the image receptor, foreshortening will occur. If the part is placed parallel to the image receptor but the central ray is angled to the image receptor, elongation will occur.

50. The correct answer is (D).

This radiograph is overexposed and any change should lead to a decrease in exposure to the patient. Setting the density control to −1 is the only choice that will lead to decreased exposure. Selecting detector C will increase the exposure because the spine lies over the detector and will be more difficult to penetrate than the lung field.

51. The correct answer is (B).

Spectral matching is the paired characteristics of a film-screen combination. To get the full benefit of a film-screen combination, the film must be sensitive to the light emitted from the screen in the cassette. If the screen and film are mismatched, an image will still appear but it will be underexposed and therefore lighter than what would be expected.

52. The correct answer is (D).

Increasing screen speed through increased intensifying screen conversion efficiency refers to the amount of light given off by the phosphors located in intensifying screens. As the conversion efficiency increases, the number of light photons given off by each phosphor also increases. This results in a decreased need for X-ray photons (radiographic technique) in order to produce an appropriate density but also means that less information is available on the image receptor (increased noise and decreased recorded detail).

53. The correct answer is (B).

Compton interactions are the primary contributors to scattered radiation. As kVp increases, the likelihood that an incident X-ray photon will interact with matter through a Compton interaction increases significantly. At low kVp settings, the percentage of Compton interactions is relatively low (around 21 percent at 50 kVp). At higher kVp settings (around 120 kVp), the percentage of Compton interactions is much higher (approximately 83 percent). This is the reason images produced at higher kVp settings exhibit reduced radiographic contrast.

54. The correct answer is (A).

When increased collimation is utilized, a smaller volume of tissue is irradiated and, therefore, less scatter is produced. Because less scatter is produced, less scatter reaches the image receptor and radiographic density is decreased. In order to maintain radiographic density when shifting from a noncollimated technique to a collimated technique, an increase in mAs is necessary to compensate.

55. The correct answer is (A).

Placing an angle on the tube (in relation to the image receptor) results in elongation of the anatomical structure. Elongation magnifies the anatomical structure unevenly and causes one end (the end farthest from the tube) to be especially magnified. Increased magnification leads to a decrease in recorded detail. Foreshortening occurs when the anatomical structure is angled to the image receptor.

56. The correct answer is (A).

The air-gap technique is used as an alternative to grids. If a space is created between the patient and the image receptor, some of the scattered radiation created inside the patient will be scattered in such a way that it will miss the image receptor and not add information to the finished image. This will increase contrast, although the increased OID will decrease recorded detail. The subtraction of some scattered radiation from the image may also slightly decrease the overall density on the finished radiograph.

57. The correct answer is (C).

In order to solve this problem, the radiographer must first know the Bucky factors (grid factors). The average grid factors are listed below:

No	Grid	1
5:1	Grid	2
8:1	Grid	4
12:1	Grid	5
16:1	Grid	6

Using these grid factors and the original mAs, use the following formula to find the new mAs:

$$\frac{mAs_1}{mAs_2} = \frac{Body\ factor_1}{Body\ factor_2}$$

$$\frac{10}{mAs_2} = \frac{4}{5}$$

Now solve for the new mAs by cross-multiplying and then dividing by the original Bucky factor:

$$mAs_2 = 50/4$$

$$mAs_2 = 12.5$$

58. The correct answer is (B).

The beam coming out of the X-ray tube is divergent—in other words, it comes out at an angle much like a flashlight beam expands as it travels from the flashlight. Because of this, the lead strips in a grid are often angled to match the angle of the X-ray beam. This allows the X-rays critical to image formation to pass through the grid without allowing the scattered radiation to reach the image receptor. For this to occur properly, the grid is designed to be used at a specific distance (focused). If the grid is moved too close or too far from the point at which it is focused, the X-rays that add to the image are absorbed by the edges of the grid. If the grid is accidentally placed upside down, the same thing occurs. When a grid is placed off center, the density is generally decreased across the entire image.

59. The correct answer is (D).

The exposure maintenance formula (also known as the direct square law) must be used to solve this problem (New mAs = Old mAs × New Distance^2/Old Distance^2). Rooted in the inverse square law, this formula follows the general rule that radiation intensity decreases to the square of the distance increase. However, instead of stating a change in radiation intensity, the exposure maintenance formula describes the change in mAs necessary to compensate for the change in distance. The exposure maintenance formula does not describe an inverse relationship; in other words, if distance increases, the mAs will also need to increase in order to compensate. To solve this problem, replace the values in the formula:

New mAs $= 25 \times 60^2/40^2$

New mAs $= 25 \times 3{,}600/1{,}600$

New mAs $= 90{,}000/1{,}600$

New mAs $= 56$

60. The correct answer is (C).

The main reason why the small focal spot should not be routinely used is that X-ray production occurs in a much smaller area when using a small focal spot than when using a large focal spot. Because many more heat interactions than X-ray interactions occur when X-rays are produced, heat can be very damaging to the anode. When a large focal spot is used, this heat is spread over a wider area and is much easier on the anode. If a large technique is desired, as in a lateral lumbar spine exam, the large focal spot should be used so that a technique can be set high enough to penetrate the anatomy. In the present case, a highly detailed image is not the goal of the exam. For a small object like a finger, though, a detailed image is desired so that the smaller anatomy can be visualized. The small focal spot should be used in this case because the technique is not high enough to strain the tube and the decreased focal spot size will increase the detail of the image.

61. The correct answer is (A).

Adding filtration and adjusting the technique to compensate has roughly the same effect as increasing the kVp and adjusting the technique to compensate: increased production of scatter, lower contrast, and a noisier image.

62. The correct answer is (D).

Quantum mottle can be defined as a noisy, grainy appearance of anatomy on a radiograph due to a low number of X-rays reaching the image receptor. This is often caused by a severe decrease in mAs brought on by a high kVp technique or a very fast intensifying screen.

63. The correct answer is (C).

The thicker an object is, the more distorted it appears on a finished radiograph. This occurs mainly because of the geometric factor of *OID*. Thicker anatomical structures are located further from the image receptor than thinner objects, such as a hand, so they are magnified to a greater degree than a smaller object would be. In addition, the surfaces of larger objects are farther apart, so the surface farthest from the image receptor appears larger than the surface located closer.

64. The correct answer is (A).

Because of the attenuation of X-rays by the anode, the cathode side of the X-ray beam is significantly stronger than the anode side. For this reason, it is wise to position the X-ray tube so that the anode is located over the thinnest part of the anatomy and the cathode is located over the thickest part. In the case of an AP femur examination, the area closer to the pelvis is thicker than the patient's knee so the cathode should be positioned on the superior side of the patient.

65. The correct answer is (C).

Patient motion remains the number one cause of motion blur. Patient communication, through the giving of clear instructions regarding breathing and movement, is the best way to reduce motion blur.

66. The correct answer is (B).

The two pictures demonstrate an exam performed with open collimation (A) and tight collimation (B). Because the X-ray beam interacts with less tissue in B, less scatter is produced, thus increasing the radiographic contrast. This will also reduce the density slightly because less scatter reaches the image receptor. Collimation does not directly affect detail and distortion.

67. The correct answer is (D).

Pediatric patients are often unwilling or unable to comply with breathing or movement instructions. Because of this, motion will often appear on a finished radiograph if the exposure time is not set at a lower value than what may typically be used for an adult. Other technical factors such as kVp and mAs should be set 25 to 50 percent lower than what would be used for adults due to the smaller size and underdevelopment of the pediatric skeletal structure.

68. The correct answer is (B).

Using a screen instead of direct film radiography significantly reduces a patient's radiation dose. When a screen is used, fewer X-ray photons are needed to create a diagnostic image and mAs can be reduced. Unfortunately, when screens are used, recorded detail decreases. This decrease in recorded detail is not immediately apparent with slow-speed screens but can become a significant problem when faster speed screens are utilized.

69. The correct answer is (D).

If the patient is in the left lateral position, the tumor will be located farther from the image receptor than in any of the other positions. This increases the *object-to-image receptor* (OID) distance, which increases the magnification.

70. The correct answer is (C).

The 15 percent rule refers to the impact of kVp on radiographic density. A relatively small increase in kVp, such as 15 percent, will cause the radiographic density to double. Answer (C) is correct because it raises kVp 15 percent and doubles the density. Answer (D) raises the kVp 15 percent as well but also increases the mAs, which is not a component of the 15 percent rule.

71. The correct answer is (A).

Direct digital radiography systems are able to convert X-radiation directly into an electronic signal without having to scan and convert photostimulable phosphor plates. This greatly shortens the image processing time but is more expensive to use since existing equipment must be replaced.

72. The correct answer is (C).

The area bordered by A contains the lung field, which consists of highly contrasting anatomical structures such as air, bone, and lung tissue. These tissues are made of different substances that *attenuate* an X-ray beam differently. The area bordered by B contains organs of the body that are very close to each other in terms of substance and attenuation. Because there is a great deal more *subject contrast* in area A, that area will display increased contrast on the finished image. Although grids and kVp affect contrast, it is highly unlikely that they could be adjusted during the exposure. The heel effect will result in variations in density across the finished image, but not to the degree shown in this example.

73. The correct answer is (C).

Most computed radiography systems are set to mimic the response a radiographer would achieve with a 200 to 400 film-screen system. Because computed radiography systems respond similarly to the way film-screen systems react, radiographic techniques used with film-screen will, on average, work well with computed radiography. Once the system is in place, the technical factors may have to be fine-tuned for specific exams. The computed radiography system can be adjusted to mimic just about any speed used with film-screen radiography.

74. The correct answer is (A).

Film-screen systems are superior to computed radiography in terms of spatial resolution—or recorded detail. The pixel size is the limiting factor for computed radiography. However, computed radiography outperforms film-screen systems in the area of contrast resolution, which is the image receptor's ability to differentiate two objects with slight variations in density. Both film-screen and computed radiography are subject to the effects of SID, OID, and angulation on size distortion.

75. The correct answer is (B).

Direct digital radiography utilizes solid-state detectors to transfer data directly to a computer, eliminating the need to use individual cassettes. This also eliminates the extra step of converting an analog image on a photostimulable phosphor plate into digital information. Other aspects of radiography, such as collimation, marking, and correctly centering, remain virtually unchanged.

76. The correct answer is (A).

If the grid ratio changes, the following grid conversion formula must be used: New mAs = Original mAs × New Grid Conversion Factor/Original Grid Conversion Factor. Since our original mAs was 40 and the New Grid's Conversion Factor is 5.5 at 85 kVp, this results in a product of 220. This number is then divided by the original conversion factor of 4 to give us the answer of 55 mAs. Although the other answers contain changes that affect density, we would not increase kVp in this case to maintain density because grids are used to improve contrast; increased kVp would degrade contrast. Also, increasing kVp by 15 percent, as is seen in this example, would increase density beyond what is needed to maintain density. Increasing SID in this example will decrease density. Focal spot size has little, if any, effect on film density.

77. The correct answer is (C).

kVp is the only factor in this question that influences contrast. Contrast is improved as kVp is reduced, so 72 kVp would produce the best contrast. Choice (D) is incorrect because a reduction in kVp without an increase in mAs will fail to maintain radiographic density.

78. The correct answer is (B).

A decrease in OID greatly improves the recorded detail on a radiograph. By turning a patient from AP to PA, the lumbar spine would be further from the image receptor and a larger OID would result. The same technique would be used regardless of AP or PA position.

79. The correct answer is (C).

Quantum mottle is caused by too few X-ray photons striking the image receptor to create the image. The only way to solve this problem is to increase mAs so that more X-ray photons will ultimately reach the image receptor.

80. The correct answer is (A).

mAs is the product of mA and time (s). The *reciprocity law* states that mAs value is the same regardless of the mA and time used to produce it. In other words, 200 mA × 0.1 seconds = 20 mAs, and 100 mA × 0.2 seconds = 20 mAs. Even though different numbers are used, the mAs values are the same and mAs will respond in the same way regardless of the values used to achieve it.

81. The correct answer is (B).

The patient's size contributes to the detail that can be seen on the finished image. In this scenario, Patient A is larger than Patient B so the anatomical structures located in Patient A are located farther from the image receptor, increasing magnification and decreasing recorded detail.

82. The correct answer is (C).

The manufacturing process determines how quickly a film will produce a density when it is exposed to X-ray or light photons. Faster films require less radiation in order to produce a density. mAs, or mA, should always be used to adjust a technique if no other change is desired. Decreasing the kVp would allow a radiographer to maintain film density, but it would also change the visible contrast on the image.

83. The correct answer is (B).

Above 80 kVp a great deal of scattered radiation is produced that will degrade the contrast on a digital image. The addition of a grid will absorb scattered radiation and improve the overall quality of the image.

84. The correct answer is (B).

Note that this question is asking for the minimum change necessary to produce a noticeable change in density. It does not take a large change in kVp to affect the density on a finished radiograph—15 percent would effectively double the amount of density. In mAs, 30 percent is the minimum change needed to produce a noticeable change in radiographic density.

85. The correct answer is (A).

Fixed, high, and automatic exposure charts normally use a higher kVp than variable kilovoltage charts. Because kVp is increased, mAs can be dramatically decreased and a savings in patient dose results. The trade-off between variable kilovoltage charts and other charts is in image quality; because variable kilovoltage charts allow for small variations in kVp, contrast is generally better. This kVp is generally the highest kVp capable of producing an acceptable quality radiograph.

86. The correct answer is (B).

By compressing anatomy through the use of a compression paddle or compression band, the radiographer is essentially reducing the volume of tissue being irradiated. Decreasing the amount of tissue means less scatter is produced, which increases radiographic contrast; and a decreased radiographic technique is required to penetrate the tissue, leading to a decreased dose to the patient. Compression will also bring anatomy closer to the image receptor, which increases recorded detail.

87. The correct answer is (C).

As the grid ratio increases, the grid's ability to remove scattered radiation and improve contrast will also improve. The grid ratio is determined by dividing the height of the grid by the thickness of the interspace material. The grid height and interspace size are listed for each of the three different grids. Grid A has a height of 5 mm and an interspace size of 1 mm, for a ratio of 5:1. Grid B has a height of 3 mm and a thickness of 0.5 mm, for a ratio of 6:1. Grid C has the highest ratio, because it has a thickness of 2 mm and an interspace size of 0.2 mm or a grid ratio of 10:1.

88. The correct answer is (A).

Because of the *divergent* nature of the X-ray beam, anatomy located further from the central ray will become more distorted. The only location on the radiographic image in which no shape distortion appears is along the path of the central ray.

89. The correct answer is (C).

The most important thing for a radiographer to do when using an automatic exposure device is to position the anatomy of interest directly above the AEC device. If the anatomy of interest is positioned to the side of the ionization chamber, the AEC device will either stay on too long or shut off prematurely, leading to an image that is either overexposed or underexposed. The AEC is capable of adapting to changes in SID. Because the AEC ultimately controls the time setting and the radiographer controls the mA and the kVp, it is not necessary for the radiographer to set the time.

90. The correct answer is (C).

A kVp setting below 80 will provide the contrast needed to outline the colon but will not be capable of penetrating the barium within the colon and allow visualization of internal structures. In order to penetrate the barium inside the colon, a setting of 90 kVp or higher is necessary.

Image Processing and Quality Assurance

1. The correct answer is (A).

Film stored at higher temperatures will age prematurely and begin to show increased density. Film can be stored below 55°F but it must be brought up to room temperature slowly to avoid condensation. Therefore, a range of 55 to 68°F is optimal for film storage.

2. The correct answer is (A).

Film should always be stored on end to avoid pressure artifacts.

3. The correct answer is (C).

If the chemicals in the developer work too efficiently, the image will exhibit an increased density across the entire film or a portion of the film. Because this increased density is the result of chemical actions, it is known as *chemical fog*. Problems in the processor, such as increased temperature and/or an increased concentration of chemicals, will cause these chemicals to do their job much too quickly and chemical fog will result.

4. The correct answer is (B).

Plus densities are areas of increased density on a finished film caused by a buildup of chemical residue, dirt, or the result of pressure or bending. Identifying a plus-density artifact will help in identifying the cause of the artifact and allow the radiographer to rule out other causes.

5. The correct answer is (A).

Small scratches at the leading and/or trailing edge of the film are most likely due to the part of the processor that guides a film from one processing tank to another (guide shoes). It is not unusual for these scratches to appear, but they should be no longer than 0.25 inch. If the scratches are longer than 0.25 inch, the crossover assemblies should be checked to make sure they are in the correct position. The direction of travel is important when identifying guide-shoe marks; the marks will always follow the direction of film travel.

6. The correct answer is (B).

The artifact shown in the illustration is called a *Pi line* due to the fact that it is the result of residue on a 1-inch roller (pi is the circumference of a 1-inch-diameter roller, or 3.14 inches). Generally, Pi lines are the result of emulsion building up on a roller until it is deposited on one or more films. It always appears perpendicular to the direction of film travel. This line can usually be wiped off the film. This artifact can be avoided altogether by cleaning the rollers regularly and replacing rollers that have become worn or rough.

7. The correct answer is (C).

Static discharge that interacts with the film results in a plus-density artifact that looks like a tree branch, a spider web, or a group of smudges. The artifact is the result of static discharge that occurs in a darkroom while the film is being handled or placed on the feed tray. Low humidity, static buildup from carpeting, or even a small charge in the feed tray may increase the appearance of static artifacts. In order to avoid this artifact, the humidity in the darkroom should be kept between 30 percent and 50 percent, antistatic mats should be used, and all equipment in the darkroom should be properly grounded.

8. The correct answer is (A).

Because radiographic images are considered part of a patient's medical record, they should be treated like any other legal document. As with all legal documents, it is important that the identification placed on the image be correct and permanently affixed. Although some departments may allow for the addition or correction of patient information with use of a permanent marker, this would not be a wise course of action for routine use. Using lead markers or light exposure (flashing) ensures that the correct patient information is attached to the radiographic image.

9. The correct answer is (C).

In the developer, black metallic silver combines with exposed silver halide crystals to create the radiographic image. Although the image becomes visible, it will quickly become fogged in normal light since the unexposed silver halide crystals have not yet been removed from the film.

10. The correct answer is (A).

Extreme changes in temperature can have negative consequences for radiographic film. In the developer and fixer, the film emulsion is relatively soft so that the chemicals can penetrate the emulsion and develop the image. It is not until the film gets to the wash and dryer that it begins to harden. If this hardening is performed too quickly, the fragile emulsion can crack and the image may be ruined.

11. The correct answer is (A).

The fixer contains a clearing agent that removes unexposed silver halide crystals from the film and sends them to the silver recovery system of the processor. If the fixer is not working properly and the undeveloped silver halide crystals are not removed, the film will have a milky appearance when it comes out of the processor. Because the silver halide crystals that are removed from the film contain real silver, it is advantageous for the department to recover and sell this silver. This is also a good practice to protect the environment.

12. The correct answer is (B).

Most of the developer chemicals have been removed by the fixer once the film reaches the wash tank, so the majority of chemicals that are removed from the film in the wash are from the fixer tank. If the fixer is not adequately removed in the wash, it will continue to slowly work on the film emulsion, and premature aging (*yellowing*) will occur. The wash water quickly becomes saturated with fixer during processing, and failures of this nature generally occur when the wash tank is not turned on, the water is not adequately agitated, or the water is circulating at a decreased rate.

13. The correct answer is (C).

The dryer does more than simply remove excess water from the processed film; it performs a vital function to protect the radiographic image. The dryer uses relatively high temperatures (120 to 150°F) to harden the film that has been softened by other chemicals to assist in the development process. Silver halide crystals are removed in the fixer.

14. The correct answer is (C).

The transportation system consists of *rollers*, *crossover networks*, and a *drive system* that moves the film all the way through the automatic processor. The drive system controls the speed with which the film travels through the processor, and thus controls how long the film spends in each individual tank of chemicals. The replenishment system adds chemicals to the tanks and the recirculation system ensures that the chemicals are properly mixed.

15. The correct answer is (C).

Chemicals called bromides that typically control the action of the developer are deposited into the tank by the emulsion of the film. During the chemical reaction that occurs during development, these bromides are removed from the emulsion and deposited in the developer solution. Since these chemicals are not present in a fresh tank of developer chemicals, a starter solution that contains bromides is added to the tank to control the action of the developer until the development process begins to add bromides during normal processing. If a starter solution is not used, the first films that run through the processor will demonstrate increased radiographic density.

16. The correct answer is (A).

Sensors located in the automatic processor are able to determine the length of a film and add the correct amount of chemicals to the tank to replace the chemicals used during development. They are generally set up for a film to be fed into the processor in a lengthwise orientation. Continuously running films crossways will deplete the amount of chemistry in the tanks and lead to underdeveloped images.

17. The correct answer is (D).

Tank A contains the developer solution, while Tank B contains the chemicals used in the fixer. The fixer chemicals are designed to stop the action of the developer chemicals; therefore, fixer chemicals in the developer would severely slow the development process. An amount as small as 10 ml of fixer solution in a 10-liter developer tank would totally stop development. Tank C contains water for the wash; small quantities of water escaping into the other tanks would not cause a problem since water is used as a solvent in the three tanks that contain chemical solutions.

18. The correct answer is (C).

Once chemicals have been added to the automatic processor, they are agitated and mixed by the circulation system in order to ensure consistent chemistry throughout the processor. Because the chemicals are in motion due to the action of the circulation system, heat from the *temperature control system* is transferred throughout the processor as well. Chemical replenishment is performed by the replenishment system.

19. The correct answer is (B).

The only indication that a film is safely in the processor is an audible beeping noise. An additional film can be placed into the automatic processor at any time, which can lead to the processor jamming or to films sticking together. If the radiographer does not wait for the beeping noise and opens the door to the darkroom or turns on a light, the film may be ruined.

20. The correct answer is (C).

Flood replenishment pumps chemicals into the processor tanks on a time interval, as opposed to *volume* replenishment that adds chemicals based on actual processor usage (number and size of films). Floor replenishment is particularly effective in low-use situations because it keeps the chemistry fresh. *Standard* (B) and *extended* (D) refer to the processor setting that controls the length of time a film will spend in the processor.

21. The correct answer is (D).

A cassette should ideally never be opened more than 2 to 3 inches while the film is removed and replaced. This will keep dust, dirt, and moisture from settling on the screen inside the cassette. Although it is a good idea to clean cassettes and intensifying screens regularly (once a week, for example), it is not necessary to clean or inspect them after *every* use. Bare hands will not damage the cassette or intensifying screens if the cassettes are cleaned regularly.

22. The correct answer is (D).

The longer the period of time that a film spends in the developer, the more the radiographic density will increase. The same is true of developer temperature; as temperature increases, the chemical activity of the developer increases and so does radiographic density. When the developer chemicals are more concentrated than required, they are able to penetrate the entire emulsion of the film and deposit metallic silver in places that were not exposed by radiation or light; this increases radiographic density.

23. The correct answer is (A).

With a daylight processor the cassette is placed directly into a slot in the front of the processor and the processor automatically opens the cassette, removes the film from the cassette, sends the exposed film for processing, places a new film into the cassette, and returns the cassette to the front of the processor for reuse. When using a daylight processor, it is not necessary for the radiographer to enter a darkroom, touch undeveloped films, or place a film on a feed tray. All other components of an automatic processor function normally.

24. The correct answer is (D).

Although marking additional information on an image is perfectly acceptable, the only item that *must* be included on every radiograph is the Right or Left identification. This identification must be placed on the image during the exposure, not afterwards with a permanent marker or even with an electronic stamp. Other information that must be included on each radiograph includes the date of the exam, the patient's identification (name or ID number), and the name of the institution.

25. The correct answer is (B).

The crossover assembly can easily become contaminated with chemical residue and emulsion deposited by films passing through. The crossover assembly should be removed, rinsed, and lightly scrubbed with a soft sponge, if necessary. The feed tray should be cleaned daily, but it is not necessary to remove the feed tray from the processor in order to perform the cleaning. The other parts of the processor listed here should be kept clean as well, but it is not necessary to clean them daily.

26. The correct answer is (C).

The developer and fixer tanks are generally drained only during the monthly cleaning cycle. The developer filter is replaced monthly as well. The lid is raised to keep chemical fumes from building up in the processor while it is not being used.

27. The correct answer is (B).

The mid-density point, or *speed indicator*, is a measurement of the speed of the entire processing system. When images are processed, it is important that the chemistry is stable so that images are consistent from day to day. The mid-density point is used in *sensitometry* (the measurement of processor performance) to indicate the ability of the processor chemistry to create an appropriate density on the finished image. If the reading is 0.10 higher than normal, the images will demonstrate increased density; conversely, if the mid-density point is 0.10 lower than normal, the image will demonstrate decreased density. A robust sensitometry program will ensure a consistent processor and good-quality images.

28. The correct answer is (D).

Section D of this illustration represents the dryer, where temperatures reach 120 to 150°F. The other sections of the automatic processor contain chemicals that maintain a temperature of 93 to 95°F.

29. The correct answer is (C).

Just as its name implies, the base + fog measurement evaluates the effect of the film base and any additional fog on the preprocessed image. The base + fog measurement also evaluates the storage conditions of film. If film becomes fogged due to radiation, light, or chemical contamination, the base + fog measurement will identify the problem. In order for the base + fog reading to be considered stable, it must be maintained between ± 0.05 of its original reading. Density difference (a) is determined by subtracting the D_{min} reading from the D_{max} measurement and is a measure of film contrast.

30. The correct answer is (B).

The archiving procedure prepares a film to be stored for several years by removing excess chemicals from the emulsion. The wash removes the residual fixer from the film so that yellowing of the film does not occur while the film is in storage. The dryer seals the emulsion and hardens the supercoat to help protect the image from scratching. The fixer is responsible for "fixing" the image permanently so that it can be viewed in white light, but the retention of fixer in the emulsion will quickly degrade the archiving quality of a radiographic image.

31. The correct answer is (A).

Resolution or recorded detail is measured in line pairs per millimeter (lp/mm). General radiographic film is capable of resolution in the range of 5 lp/mm, although mammography film can exceed 5 lp/mm. The resolution of digital imaging is much less than that of film, although its ability to increase quality in other areas makes it the imaging system of choice for many radiography departments.

32. The correct answer is (D).

Pixels are the *picture elements* of a digital image that are extremely tiny squares comprised of a various shades of gray—all the way from white to black. The image itself is made of thousands of individual pixels that blend together to form the digital image. The matrix size indicates how many pixels are located within the viewing area. Therefore, if the viewing size remains constant (the screen size on a monitor, for example) and the matrix size increases (more total pixels), the size of the pixels will have to decrease. The smaller the pixel size, the better the image resolution.

33. The correct answer is (B).

Window *width* controls image contrast inversely: as the window width is increased, the overall contrast decreases. The window *level* controls density directly: as the window level increases, density increases.

34. The correct answer is (D).

Storing images electronically allows them to be copied and stored at multiple locations so that if there is a disaster at one location (fire, flood, etc.), the images will remain intact at another location. The ability to send images electronically provides the additional benefit of allowing multiple users to view the images at separate sites. Also, images can be sent quickly to various locations, which may take hours or days with a film-based archiving system.

35. The correct answer is (B).

DICOM stands for *Digital Imaging COmmunication in Medicine*; it was designed in the early 1990s by the American College of Radiology and the National Electrical Manufacturers Association (NEMA). Through the use of the DICOM "language," every piece of digital imaging equipment can interact with every other piece; more importantly, every piece of equipment can also interact with the storage system so that images from all modalities can be stored in the same system and can be retrieved to any modality as needed. The other two answers in this question refer to a test pattern used for digital imaging (SMPTE, Society of Motion Picture and Television Engineers) and software used to link patient information and images in a radiology department (RIS, Radiology Information System).

36. The correct answer is (B).

Photostimulable phosphor plates create a latent image by "capturing" *energy* in the phosphor layer. This energy will dissipate over time and degrade the finished image if the processing does not occur in a timely manner. One-fourth of the image is lost after 8 hours, and the image will continue to lose energy until almost all of it is gone after just a few days.

Criteria for Image Evaluation

1. The correct answer is (A).

mAs is the controlling factor of radiographic density because density increases as mAs increases and decreases as mAs decreases. Although an increase as small as 30 percent in mAs will result in a visible change in density, a change of 100 percent (a doubling of mAs or an increase by a factor of 2) is necessary to adequately change mAs.

2. The correct answer is (C).

Grids are used to clean up the scattered radiation that is produced by the patient during an exposure. Because scattered radiation degrades the contrast on an image, much better radiographic contrast will be demonstrated on a film produced with a grid than on a film produced without a grid.

3. The correct answer is (B).

Poor film/screen contact will create a small area of unsharpness on a finished film but will rarely cause a loss of detail across the entire image. The cause of poor film/screen contact is worn or warped screens, or residue in between the film and screen that prevents the film and the screen from making direct contact with each other during the exposure. The other answer choices would all cause unsharpness across the entire film, but not in only one area.

4. The correct answer is (C).

The kidneys lie near the patient's back, so performing a PA abdomen will position the kidneys farther from the image receptor than what would be seen in an AP abdominal radiograph. Because increasing the OID increases the amount of size distortion, the kidneys will appear larger in the PA radiograph. Performing the exam PA will also increase the amount of size distortion and decrease the detail seen in the spine—the opposite of answer (D). Contrast and density are not noticeably changed by positioning a patient AP or PA.

5. The correct answer is (C).

Magnification occurs on every radiograph because it is never possible to place an anatomical part directly on an image receptor. Elongation will occur if the central ray is off target because the beam will act as if it is angled across the anatomy. Foreshortening is reduced if the central ray is directed perpendicular to the anatomy of interest.

6. The correct answer is (B).

Every radiograph has to clearly identify which portion of the anatomy is right or left. This marking must occur on the radiographic image and not be written or flashed onto the image after exposure. Correctly marking right or left protects the patient and ensures that procedures will be completed on the correct anatomical part. Other markers may be added as needed, but right or left markers must appear on all radiographs.

7. The correct answer is (B).

Voluntary muscle movement includes all skeletal muscles used for movement as well as the muscles involved in breathing. If a patient moves or breathes during an exposure, motion will be seen on the entire radiograph. If the motion is due to involuntary muscle movement, the motion will be seen only in the localized area where the motion takes place: in the digestive system, generally as a result of peristalsis, or in the chest due to the movement of the heart. Poor film-screen contact is localized in one area or several small areas of an image. Image processing will not cause blurring of the image.

8. The correct answer is (A).

Grids are made of alternating strips of lead and an interspace material. Because the lead strips attenuate a portion of the X-ray beam, they can sometimes be seen on a completed radiograph. Although the processor can cause lines on a completed image, there will not be hundreds of them, and they will generally appear more prominent than grid lines. The lines seen on a radiograph due to static discharge will appear random, not parallel.

9. The correct answer is (D).

A cracked safelight filter will allow unfiltered (white) light to escape from the safelight and strike the film, causing an increase in density across the film. Choices (A) and (B) in this question would result in light films, and choice (C) would result in white specks on a completed image.

10. The correct answer is (C).

Noise is the grainy appearance caused by decreased mAs and is the result of high kVp techniques or very fast screen speeds. Because of the decrease in mAs, an insufficient number of X-rays are available to produce a quality image.

11. The correct answer is (B).

Increasing distance without making any other change will decrease radiographic density on a finished image. In the two illustrations, Configuration A is closer to an image receptor than Configuration B, so greater density will occur with Configuration A if the same technique is utilized. Configuration B will result in increased detail due to the longer SID as well as decreased patient dose. Distance does not affect motion blur.

12. The correct answer is (B).

kVp is a primary controller of the contrast seen on a radiographic image. By decreasing kVp and increasing mAs, less scatter will be produced, contrast will improve, and radiographic density will remain unchanged. The changes in choices (C) and (D) would maintain density but not significantly affect contrast.

13. The correct answer is (D).

If time is decreased and mA is increased, the image will not be affected because mAs remains the same. This is called the *reciprocity law*. Choice (A) would lead to decreased contrast, and choices (B) and (C) would lead to decreased radiographic detail.

14. The correct answer is (C).

Increasing the OID without adjusting SID will increase magnification on the completed image. Observation of the four images in this question shows that the greatest magnification is demonstrated on Image C (most notably, the femurs are clipped on Image C).

15. The correct answer is (A).

The reason for placing an angle on the central ray is to reduce the superimposition of the clavicle over the scapula and superior ribs. Although the angle allows for greater demonstration of the clavicle, the image will appear more distorted. Magnification will occur to the same or greater degree than that seen on the AP projection.

16. The correct answer is (B).

No patient identification information is seen on this radiograph. This information may be added after exposure but must be placed on the image prior to processing (with the use of a *flasher*, for example). The other information that is missing on this radiograph is the name of the institution. Adding the technologist's name or initials is not always necessary but is a good way to determine who is responsible for the image.

17. The correct answer is (C).

Paget disease is an additive condition that is caused by an increase in bone growth. Because more bone tissue is present than what would be expected, the resulting image would be underexposed if a normal technique is used. In order to compensate for the increase in bone tissue, the radiographic technique must be increased.

18. The correct answer is (A).

Crescent marks like the one shown in the image are caused by the film being bent prior to processing.

19. The correct answer is (D).

Film that has been stored for a long period of time will begin to lose its ability to function as it was designed to, and will lose both speed and contrast. Because expired film has been stored for a long period of time, it will become fogged by light, radiation, and chemical fumes. This will add a slight density to the film that will additionally degrade radiographic contrast but not be sufficient to increase density beyond what is normally anticipated.

20. The correct answer is (D).

Noise is the "grainy" appearance of an image caused by a mAs setting that is far too low to provide enough information to provide a quality image. Image A displays decreased contrast, Image B displays increased density, and Image C displays increased contrast.

21. The correct answer is (A).

Use of a 10-foot distance will increase radiographic detail and decrease magnification. The reduced magnification helps to ensure that all of the desired anatomy (the costophrenic angles, for example) will be displayed on the completed image. Increasing SID requires that mAs be increased, however, which may lead to greater exposure times and an increased possibility of motion artifacts.

22. The correct answer is (B).

Radiation fog is caused by scattered radiation striking the stored film in the exam room. Film should be stored in a darkroom or a storage facility that is free of scatter radiation. Chemical fog (A) is a by-product of a poorly maintained processor. Temperature fog (C) is a result of increased storage temperature or increased temperature in the processor. Fog from a safelight (D) occurs in the darkroom and is the result of a cracked or damaged safelight filter.

23. The correct answer is (D).

The distinct characteristic of static discharge is the branching artifact seen on the left side of the artifact. The central portion of the artifact is caused by static as well. A pressure artifact (A) or poor film-screen contact (C) will appear less distinct and blurry. Dirt in a cassette will appear as a minus density (white) rather than a plus density, as seen in this image.

24. The correct answer is (A).

Osteoporosis is a destructive disease that weakens or thins bone; if technique is not reduced, the resulting image will display increased density. The other pathological conditions listed in the question would all require an increase in technique in order to maintain radiographic density.

Chapter 7: **Radiation Protection**

Biologic Aspects of Radiation

1. Which of the following cells is the most radio-sensitive?

   (A) Fibroblast
   (B) Lymphocyte
   (C) Myocyte
   (D) Neuron

2. A reaction is produced by 5 Gy of a test radiation. It takes 25 Gy of 250 kVp X-rays to produce this reaction. Which of the following is the relative biologic effectiveness of the test radiation?

   RBE

   (A) 0.25
   (B) 5
   (C) 10
   (D) 25

3. During an accident at a nuclear facility 1 month ago, an individual received a radiation dose of 3 Gy (300 rad). Which of the following is the most appropriate measure of radiation lethality?

   (A) LD$_{10/20}$
   (B) LD$_{50/30}$
   (C) LD$_{50/60}$ 300/30
   (D) LD$_{100/60}$

       10/1

4. An employee of a radiologic facility is diagnosed with cataracts after 25 years of employment. Which of the following are also late somatic effects of radiation?

   1. Cancer
   2. Erythema
   3. Life-span shortening

   (A) 1 only
   (B) 2 only
   (C) 1 and 2 only
   (D) 1 and 3 only

5. A 33-year-old male patient has an abdominal X-ray performed. He is concerned about radiation exposure–induced sterility. Which of the following doses can result in permanent sterility?

   (A) 0.1 Gy
   (B) 5 Gy   1 Gy = 100 Rad
   (C) 10 rad   5 = 500
   (D) 200 rad

6. Which of the following are characteristics of radiation-induced cancer?

   1. It can be distinguished from non-radiation-induced cancer by appearance.
   2. It is an early somatic effect of radiation.
   3. It is a stochastic effect of radiation.

   (A) 1 only
   (B) 2 only
   (C) 3 only
   (D) 1, 2, and 3

KAPLAN

7. Which of the following accurately describe the dose-response relationship involved in cataractogenesis?

    1. Linear-quadratic, nonthreshold curve
    2. Linear, threshold curve
    3. Nonlinear, threshold curve

   (A) 1 only

   (B) 2 only

   (C) 3 only

   (D) 1, 2, and 3

8. A radiation worker who was inadvertently exposed to a large dose of ionizing radiation three days ago presents with nausea, fever, and patchy hair loss on his arms. Which of the following is an acute somatic effect of radiation?

   (A) Cancer

   (B) Cataracts

   (C) Erythema

   (D) Life-span shortening

9. Which of the following syndromes is most likely to occur in patients exposed to ionizing radiation doses of more than 5,000 rad?

   (A) Cardiovascular system syndrome

   (B) Central nervous system syndrome

   (C) Hematologic syndrome

   (D) Hepatic syndrome

10. Following high-dose radiation exposure, a patient develops hematological abnormalities. Which of the following cells has likely been affected?

    (A) Astrocytes

    (B) Lymphocytes

    (C) Myocytes

    (D) Oligodendrocytes

11. Which of the following are examples of effects of radiation on the skin?

    1. Desquamation
    2. Epilation
    3. Erythema

    (A) 1 only

    (B) 2 only

    (C) 1 and 2 only

    (D) 1, 2, and 3

12. Hours after an ionizing exposure to 4,000 rad, a patient develops nausea, vomiting, and diarrhea. These symptoms are consistent with which of the following syndromes?

    (A) Central nervous system syndrome

    (B) Gastrointestinal syndrome

    (C) Hematologic syndrome

    (D) Renal syndrome

13. The fetus is most susceptible to radiation-induced congenital abnormalities during which of the following stages?

    (A) 0 to 9 days

    (B) 10 days to 6 weeks

    (C) 6 weeks to term

    (D) Delivery to age 1

14. Which of the following terms is used to describe the impact of gonadal dose across the entire population?

    (A) Bone-marrow dose

    (B) Entrance skin exposure

    (C) Genetically significant dose

    (D) Relative biologic effectiveness

GO ON TO THE NEXT PAGE

15. Which of the following are characteristics of gonadal shielding?

1. It may be used in place of an adequately collimated beam.
2. It is a secondary protective measure.
3. It should be used if the testes or ovaries are within 5 cm of the X-ray beam.

(A) 1 only
(B) 2 only
(C) 1 and 2 only
(D) 2 and 3 only

Refer to the following graph for Question 16:

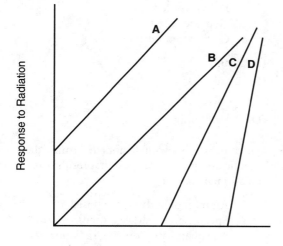

Radiation Dose

16. Which of the following (Lines A through D) represent a linear, nonthreshold relationship?

(A) Lines A and B
(B) Lines A and C
(C) Lines B and C
(D) Lines B and D

17. Which of the following statements characterizes the law of Bergonie and Tribondeau?

(A) It describes the ratio of the radiation dose that results in a biologic response.
(B) Most cells are likely to undergo programmed cell death.
(C) Pluripotent cells are among the most radiosensitive.
(D) Stochastic effects of radiation include cataract formation and carcinogenesis.

18. What is the term used to describe the programmed cell death that occurs as a result of the cellular effect of radiation?

(A) Apoptosis
(B) Direct action
(C) Point mutation
(D) Single strand break

19. Which of the following factors increases cellular radiosensitivity?

(A) Anoxia
(B) High LET
(C) Hypoxia
(D) Low LET

20. Which of the following is a process that involves the breakdown of a water molecule to produce ions and free radicals?

(A) Direct action
(B) Indirect action
(C) Linear energy transfer
(D) Target theory

21. Which of the following is the stage of the cell cycle that corresponds to DNA synthesis?

(A) G_1
(B) G_2
(C) Prophase
(D) S

GO ON TO THE NEXT PAGE

KAPLAN)

Refer to the following figures for Question 22:

Figure 1

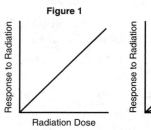

Figure 2

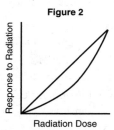

Figure 3

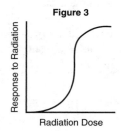

Figure 4

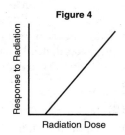

22. Which of the graphs above represents a linear, nonthreshold curve that would be used to delineate the dose-response relationship of a patient with radiation-induced leukemia?

(A) Figure 1

(B) Figure 2

(C) Figure 3

(D) Figure 4

23. Which of the following concepts are used to understand how the effects of radiation vary in biologic tissue?

   1. Linear energy transfer
   2 Oxygen enhancement ratio
   3. Target theory

(A) 1 only

(B) 2 only

(C) 1 and 2 only

(D) 2 and 3 only

24. According to the concept of genetically significant dose (GSD), a population of 600 individuals (Group A) was exposed to 0.005 Sv of gonadal radiation, and a population of 60 (Group B) was exposed to 0.05 Sv of gonadal radiation. Which of the following would be the genetic effect?

(A) The genetic effect on Group A is greater.

(B) The genetic effect on Group B is greater.

(C) The genetic effect on Group B is less.

(D) The genetic effect is equal in both groups.

25. After receiving a lethal dose of ionizing radiation, which of the following cells will have the highest rate of recovery?

   1. Deoxygenated cells
   2. Hypoxic cells
   3. Oxygenated cells

(A) 1 only

(B) 2 only

(C) 3 only

(D) 2 and 3 only

26. Which of the following factors determine the somatic and genetic damage that result from radiation exposure?

   1. Amount of body area exposed
   2. Specific body parts exposed
   3. The quantity of ionizing radiation

(A) 1 only

(B) 1 and 2 only

(C) 2 and 3 only

(D) 1, 2, and 3

GO ON TO THE NEXT PAGE

27. Ionizing radiation with a high linear energy transfer can cause biologic changes. Which of the following is an example of high LET radiation?

    (A) Alpha particles

    (B) Cosmic rays

    (C) Gamma rays

    (D) X-rays

28. Which of the following molecules is most likely to produce free radicals as a result of interaction with ionizing radiation?

    (A) Enzyme

    (B) Fat

    (C) Protein

    (D) Water

Minimizing Patient Exposure

1. What factors are affected when the radiologist uses intermittent or pulse fluoroscopy?

    1. Life of the fluoroscopic tube decreases.
    2. Life of the fluoroscopic tube increases.
    3. Patient dose decreases.

    (A) 1 only

    (B) 2 only

    (C) 1 and 3 only

    (D) 2 and 3 only

2. During a trauma, a grid is not available for a cross-table lateral cervical spine. What other factors can a radiographer use to perform the exam?

    (A) Air-gap technique

    (B) Do not perform the exam

    (C) Perform an AP cervical spine X-ray

    (D) Stand the patient up for a lateral cervical spine film

Refer to the following illustrations for Question 3

A

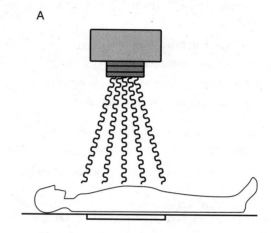

B

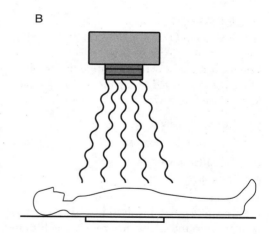

3. Figures A and B above both produce the same diagnostic image; however, which of the following will result in a high absorbed dose?

    (A) Figure A

    (B) Figure B

    (C) Figures A and B

    (D) None of the above

GO ON TO THE NEXT PAGE

KAPLAN

4. What factor is affected when the radiographer switches from a 200 to 400 film-screen combination?

   (A) Exposure time increases.
   (B) Patient exposure decreases.
   (C) Radiographic contrast is unchanged.
   (D) Radiographic density increases.

5. What are the advantages of implementing a repeat analysis program in a radiologic facility?

   1. An analysis program is not beneficial to the department.
   2. Increases alertness during image review
   3. Increases cognizance among staff and students to generate quality images

   (A) 1 only
   (B) 2 only
   (C) 1 and 2 only
   (D) 2 and 3 only

6. The most direct way to determine the amount of exposure received by a patient during a radiologic procedure is which of the following?

   (A) Bone-marrow dose
   (B) Entrance skin exposure
   (C) Gonadal dose
   (D) Skin dose

7. A pregnant woman involved in a car accident is brought into the emergency room. The ER physician suspects a cervical spine injury and needs to rule out fracture. In this situation, what protocols must the radiographer observe?

   1. Collimate to the area of interest.
   2. Provide adequate abdominal and gonadal shielding.
   3. Use the lowest exposure factors to produce a diagnostic film.

   (A) 1 only
   (B) 2 only
   (C) 2 and 3 only
   (D) 1, 2, and 3

8. Which of the following procedures generates the highest radiation dose to the patient?

   (A) AP chest radiograph
   (B) Lateral cervical spine radiograph
   (C) Lumbar spine radiograph
   (D) Small bowel series

9. Involuntary motion can result in an inadequate diagnostic film. Which of the following is an example of involuntary motion?

   (A) Breathing
   (B) Coughing
   (C) Heartbeat
   (D) Laughing

10. Emphysema is considered to be a destructive pathology. While acquiring a chest X-ray on a patient with emphysema, what should the radiographer consider?

    (A) Decreasing technique
    (B) Decreasing distance
    (C) Increasing technique
    (D) Leave technique unchanged

11. The main of objective of the radiographer is to reduce patient dose. If an exposure produces 12 mrem at 1 second, what will the new exposure be if the time is reduced to 0.50 seconds (distance is kept the same)?

    (A) 3 mrem
    (B) 6 mrem
    (C) 24 mrem
    (D) 60 mrem

12. Which device can be used to control the size of the X-ray field during an exposure?

    (A) Bucky tray
    (B) Collimator
    (C) Geiger-Müller detector
    (D) Grid

GO ON TO THE NEXT PAGE

13. In terms of patient exposure, what is the advantage of performing an abdominal radiograph in the PA projection?

    (A) Gonadal dose is decreased.
    (B) Object-to-image distance (OID) is decreased.
    (C) Radiographic contrast is increased.
    (D) Technique is decreased.

14. Which of the following devices is manufactured within the X-ray cassette and minimizes patient radiation exposure?

    (A) Emulsion
    (B) Intensifying screens
    (C) Silver halide crystals
    (D) X-ray film

15. A radiograph of the left hand was acquired. The careless technologist neglected to indicate the anatomic site of interest. This will result in which of the following?

    1. Decreased patient dose
    2. Increased patient dose
    3. Repeat radiographs

    (A) 1 only
    (B) 2 only
    (C) 1 and 3 only
    (D) 2 and 3 only

16. Which of the following are benefits of the use of image intensification fluoroscopy?

    1. Increased image brightness
    2. Patient dose reduction
    3. Smaller objects can be adequately visualized.

    (A) 1 only
    (B) 2 only
    (C) 1 and 2 only
    (D) 1, 2, and 3

17. X-ray beam limitation devices reduce patient exposure. Which of the following is a beam limitation device?

    (A) Bucky
    (B) Cone
    (C) Filter
    (D) X-ray tube

18. The amount of filtration that is required depends on the kilovoltage of the X-ray. What is the total filtration needed for a unit that operates above 70 kVp?

    (A) 1.5 mm/Al
    (B) 2.3 mm/Al
    (C) 2.5 mm/Al
    (D) 3.0 mm/Al

19. Where should a flat contact shield be placed during a fluoroscopic examination?

    (A) On the patient
    (B) To the left of the patient
    (C) To the right of the patient
    (D) Under the patient

20. An AP film of the spine in a patient with suspected scoliosis was ordered. In this instance, which type of shielding would be most effective in minimizing patient exposure?

    1. Clear lead shield
    2. Shaped contact shield
    3. Shadow shield

    (A) 1 only
    (B) 1 and 2 only
    (C) 2 and 3 only
    (D) 1, 2, and 3

GO ON TO THE NEXT PAGE

KAPLAN

21. Which of the following devices is used for the radiologic imaging of body parts with variable thickness?

    (A) Aperture diaphragm

    (B) Collimator

    (C) Compensating filter

    (D) Lead shield

22. While selecting appropriate exposure factors for an examination, which of the following should be considered?

    1. Film-screen combination
    2. Quantity of filtration
    3. Source-to-image distance (SID)

    (A) 1 only

    (B) 1 and 2 only

    (C) 2 and 3 only

    (D) 1, 2, and 3

23. Of the following devices, which absorbs scatter radiation and is made of sections with radiopaque material alternated with radiolucent material?

    (A) Bucky

    (B) Grid

    (C) Lead shielding

    (D) X-ray tube

24. While performing a fluoroscopic procedure with a stationary tube, the source-to-skin distance must not be less than which of the following?

    (A) 12 cm

    (B) 30 cm

    (C) 38 cm

    (D) 40 cm

25. Which of the following would be considered an adequate reason to order a chest X-ray?

    1. As part of a pre-employment physical
    2. For a patient admitted for treatment of a pulmonary disease
    3. To screen for tuberculosis

    (A) 1 only

    (B) 2 only

    (C) 1 and 2 only

    (D) 2 and 3 only

26. Which of the following imaging procedures will increase the technologist's risk of exposure?

    (A) C-arm fluoroscopy

    (B) General fluoroscopy

    (C) General radiographic examinations

    (D) Mobile radiography

27. During a fluoroscopic examination in the operating room, an audible signal is heard from the unit. How long does it take for the audible signal on the fluoroscopy unit to alert the radiographer?

    (A) 1 minute

    (B) 5 minutes

    (C) 15 minutes

    (D) 30 minutes

28. Which of the following is the result of a lack of communication between the radiographer and the patient?

    1. An uncooperative patient
    2. Increased patient exposure
    3. Repeat radiographs

    (A) 1 only

    (B) 1 and 2 only

    (C) 2 and 3 only

    (D) 1, 2, and 3

GO ON TO THE NEXT PAGE

29. Which of the following is an advantage of beam filtration?

    1. Increases beam quality ("hardens" the beam)
    2. Reduces exposure to the patient's skin
    3. Removes low-energy photons

  (A) 1 only

  (B) 1 and 2 only

  (C) 2 and 3 only

  (D) 1, 2, and 3

30. While acquiring a radiograph, why is it important to limit the beam to the area of interest?

    1. To prevent unnecessary exposure
    2. To reduce scatter radiation
    3. To reduce the amount of absorbed radiation

  (A) 1 only

  (B) 1 and 2 only

  (C) 2 and 3 only

  (D) 1, 2, and 3

31. A 75-year-old male patient presents to the physician with a suspected pleural effusion. On examination, fluid is noted in the right costophrenic angle. A chest X-ray is ordered to evaluate this finding. The radiograph is acquired by selecting an appropriate kVp, lateral radiation sensing cells, and a density setting of +1. Which of the following technologic features was used to acquire this chest X-ray?

  (A) Automatic exposure control

  (B) Automatic brightness control

  (C) Automatically programmed radiography

  (D) Dead-man switch

32. Which of the following grid ratios will incur the highest patient dose?

  (A) 6:1

  (B) 8:1

  (C) 10:1

  (D) 16:1

Personnel Protection

1. Protective apparel is provided to radiologic personnel to reduce occupational exposure. These devices are required to meet NCRP regulations. How often should the lead apron be imaged for cracks and leaks?

  (A) Daily

  (B) Weekly

  (C) Every 3 months

  (D) Yearly

2. Which of the following is considered a basic method of radiation protection that the technologist can employ to reduce exposure?

    1. Distance
    2. Shielding
    3. Time

  (A) 1 only

  (B) 2 only

  (C) 2 and 3 only

  (D) 1, 2, and 3

3. Which of the following protective barriers is located parallel to the X-ray beam and shields against both leakage and scatter radiation?

    1. Control booth barrier
    2. Primary protective barrier
    3. Secondary protective barrier

  (A) 1 only

  (B) 2 only

  (C) 3 only

  (D) 1 and 3 only

GO ON TO THE NEXT PAGE

KAPLAN

4. Which of the following administrative measures should be applied to reduce radiation exposure to health care personnel?

   (A) An additional dosimeter should be provided to all personnel.

   (B) Detailed records of number of examinations performed should be maintained.

   (C) One day off during the week should be scheduled.

   (D) Radiographers should be rotated through various modalities.

5. A mobile X-ray of the abdomen, forearm, and pelvis were ordered for a patient. Which of these studies will cause the most scatter?

   (A) Abdomen

   (B) Forearm

   (C) Pelvis

   (D) Scatter is equal in all films.

6. If the distance is doubled, the intensity will

   (A) decrease by a factor of 4.

   (B) increase by a factor of 2.

   (C) increase by a factor of 4.

   (D) remain the same.

7. While maneuvering a C-arm fluoroscopic tube during a hip replacement in the operating room, where should the radiographer stand?

   (A) Behind the surgeon

   (B) On the image intensifier side

   (C) On the X-ray tube side

   (D) Outside the operating room

8. What factors should be taken into consideration before designing a radiation barrier for a particular X-ray room?

   1. Occupancy factor
   2. Use factor
   3. Workload

   (A) 1 only

   (B) 2 only

   (C) 3 only

   (D) 1, 2, and 3

9. Which type of radiation generated in the X-ray tube is always present when the radiographic tube is on?

   (A) Fluoroscopic radiation

   (B) Leakage radiation

   (C) Primary radiation

   (D) Scatter radiation

10. It is important to notify the surrounding personnel while attaining a mobile radiograph. This will serve to reduce scatter radiation. Which of the following will result in the most scatter radiation?

    (A) Bucky

    (B) Cassette

    (C) Patient

    (D) X-ray tube

11. During a barium enema examination, a protective curtain should be placed between the physician and the patient. What is the minimum lead equivalent required for the curtain?

    (A) 0.25 mm Pb

    (B) 0.35 mm Pb

    (C) 0.50 mm Pb

    (D) 1.0 mm Pb

GO ON TO THE NEXT PAGE

12. A radiographer receives an order form to perform a mobile X-ray. Which of the following factors should be utilized to reduce personnel exposure?

    1. Decreased shielding
    2. Increased distance
    3. Increased exposure rate

    (A) 1 only
    (B) 2 only
    (C) 3 only
    (D) 1 and 3 only

13. Federal standards limit exposure rates of general fluoroscopy to a maximum of which of the following?

    (A) 5 R/min
    (B) $5 \times 2.58 \times 10^{-4}$ C/kg/min
    (C) 10 R/min
    (D) 20 R/min

14. Which of the following devices uses an audible signal to alert the radiographer that 5 minutes of fluoroscopy has elapsed?

    (A) Cumulative timer
    (B) Electronic timer
    (C) Exposure timer
    (D) mAs timer

15. Which of the following is a characteristic(s) of the Bucky slot cover?

    1. It must be 0.25 mm Al equivalent.
    2. It must be 0.25 mm Pb equivalent.
    3. It reduces gonadal dose.

    (A) 1 only
    (B) 2 only
    (C) 1 and 3 only
    (D) 2 and 3 only

16. Gonadal shielding should be used on both female and male patients for which of the following examinations?

    (A) AP pelvis
    (B) AP sacrum-coccyx
    (C) KUB
    (D) Lateral hip

17. A pediatric patient is brought into the hospital with a suspected right hip fracture. An AP film of the right hip is ordered. Due to the patient's age, his mother is asked to hold him. Where should the radiographer place the mother, in reference to the primary beam, to reduce her exposure?

    (A) At the end of the table
    (B) At the head of the table
    (C) On the patient's left side
    (D) On the patient's right side

18. Which of the following is an example of a primary barrier?

    (A) Control booth
    (B) Door of the X-ray suite
    (C) Lead apron
    (D) Walls of the X-ray suite (more than 7 feet in height)

GO ON TO THE NEXT PAGE

KAPLAN

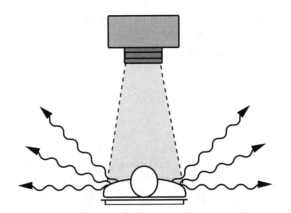

19. Using the diagram above, select the type of scatter that occurs when X-rays interact with an object.

    1. Coherent scatter
    2. Compton scatter
    3. Photoelectric effect

(A) 1 only
(B) 2 only
(C) 1 and 2 only
(D) 2 and 3 only

20. Which of the following are components of the general fluoroscopic unit?

    1. Cumulative timer
    2. Exposure switch
    3. Protective curtain

(A) 1 only
(B) 1 and 2 only
(C) 2 and 3 only
(D) 1, 2, and 3

Radiation Exposure and Monitoring

1. During an examination, a radiologist's hands are required to be near the X-ray field. In this case, which of the following monitors should he wear?

(A) Extremity dosimeter
(B) Film badge
(C) Lead gloves
(D) Thermoluminescent dosimeter

2. What is the cumulative occupational dose limit?

(A) 5 mSv/year × age in years
(B) 10 mSv/year × age in years
(C) 15 mSv/year × age in years
(D) 25 mSv/year × age in years

3. Which of the following is used to express occupational exposure?

(A) Gray
(B) rad
(C) rem
(D) Sievert

4. Results from the personnel monitoring reports should be maintained to meet both state and federal regulations. Which of the following is found on a personnel monitoring report?

    1. Cumulative dose equivalent for the past 6 months
    2. Dose-equivalent data from the first day of the month to the last
    3. Type of dosimeter used

(A) 1 only
(B) 1 and 2 only
(C) 2 and 3 only
(D) 1, 2, and 3

GO ON TO THE NEXT PAGE ⟶

5. Which of the following dosimeters resembles a fountain pen and is most useful to the health care worker who is likely to receive a high exposure to ionizing radiation over a short period of time?

   (A) Extremity dosimeter
   (B) Film badge
   (C) Pocket dosimeter
   (D) Thermal luminescent dosimeter

6. A professional weight lifter who receives a lumbar spine X-ray inquires about his daily exposure to radiation. Which of the following is the annual effective dose limit for members of the general public?

   1. 5 mSv
   2. 5 rem
   3. 50 mSv

   (A) 1 only
   (B) 2 only
   (C) 1 and 3 only
   (D) 2 and 3 only

7. A radiation survey instrument is used to detect and measure radiation. Which of the following requirements must be met prior to the use of such an instrument?

   1. It must measure cumulative radiation intensity.
   2. It should be cost effective.
   3. It should be durable enough to withstand normal use.

   (A) 1 only
   (B) 1 and 2 only
   (C) 2 and 3 only
   (D) 1, 2, and 3

8. As part of her clinical education requirement, a female radiography student rotates through a hospital for clinical training. Which of the following represents her annual effective dose limit?

   (A) 0.05 rem
   (B) 0.1 rem
   (C) 1.5 rem
   (D) 5 rem

9. Once her pregnancy has been declared, the female radiographer can continue to practice routine radiography. However, certain protocols must be observed to ensure the safety of both the mother and embryo-fetus. Which of the following is a safety measure that should be taken by the imaging facility?

   1. A second personal dosimeter should be issued to the radiographer.
   2. A separate monthly report that tracks the exposure to the radiographer and embryo-fetus must be recorded.
   3. The technologist should receive proper counseling from the radiation safety officer.

   (A) 1 only
   (B) 1 and 2 only
   (C) 2 and 3 only
   (D) 1, 2, and 3

10. What is the cumulative occupational dose for a radiographer who is 27 years old?

   (A) 10 mSv
   (B) 15 mSv
   (C) 50 mSv
   (D) 270 mSv

GO ON TO THE NEXT PAGE

KAPLAN

11. Roentgen is the unit of measure for exposure. Which of the following mathematical expressions can be used to obtain exposure?

    1. Absorbed dose × quality factor
    2. Exposure rate × time
    3. Rad × quality factor

    (A) 1 only

    (B) 2 only

    (C) 1 and 2 only

    (D) 1 and 3 only

12. Which of the following is the international system (SI) unit for radiation absorbed dose?

    (A) Coulomb per kilogram

    (B) Gray

    (C) Roentgen

    (D) Sievert

13. A nurse was issued a dosimeter while taking part in an interventional study. She inquired about the exposure received during the examination. Which of the following dosimeters provides an immediate readout of radiation exposure?

    (A) Film badge

    (B) Optically stimulated luminescence dosimeter

    (C) Pocket dosimeter

    (D) Thermoluminescent dosimeter

14. Which of the following is a product of absorbed dose and the quality factor?

    (A) Dose equivalent

    (B) Linear energy transfer

    (C) Occupancy factor

    (D) Radiation absorbed dose

15. Health care workers exposed to ionizing radiation should wear a personal dosimeter during routine radiographic procedures. Which of the following are a benefits of such a device?

    1. It is evidence of the work habits of the technologist.
    2. It is indicative of the working conditions in the facility.
    3. It provides a record of the number of exams the radiographer has completed.

    (A) 1 only

    (B) 1 and 2 only

    (C) 2 and 3 only

    (D) 1, 2, and 3

16. Which of the following instruments should be used to monitor an area that has been contaminated with radioactive material?

    (A) Dosimeter

    (B) Geiger-Müller (G-M) detector

    (C) Ionization chamber-type survey meter

    (D) Proportional counter

17. Which of the following should the radiologist wear while performing a fluoroscopic examination?

    1. Extremity dosimeter
    2. Lead apron
    3. Thyroid shield

    (A) 1 only

    (B) 1 and 2 only

    (C) 2 and 3 only

    (D) 1, 2, and 3

GO ON TO THE NEXT PAGE ▷

KAPLAN

18. Which of the following gas-filled radiation survey instruments is not useful for diagnostic imaging facilities?

    (A) Geiger-Müller (G-M) detector

    (B) Ionization chamber-type survey meter

    (C) Optically stimulated luminescence dosimeter

    (D) Proportional counter

19. According to the ALARA concept, which of the following are the cardinal principles of radiation protection?

    1. Maximizing distance
    2. Maximizing shielding
    3. Minimizing time

    (A) 1 only

    (B) 1 and 2 only

    (C) 2 and 3 only

    (D) 1, 2, and 3

20. Which of the following are advantages of a thermal luminescent dosimeter, compared to the film badge?

    1. It can be worn for up to 1 month.
    2. It is not affected by humidity, pressure, or temperature changes.
    3. LiF crystals can be reused after a reading is obtained.

    (A) 1 only

    (B) 2 only

    (C) 1 and 3 only

    (D) 2 and 3 only

Answers and Explanations

Biologic Aspects of Radiation

1. The correct answer is (B).

The highly sensitive cell types include the erythroblast, intestinal crypt cell, lymphocyte, and spermatogonia. The fibroblast (A) has an intermediate level of radiosensitivity. The myocyte (C) and neuron (D) are the least sensitive to radiation.

2. The correct answer is (B).

The relative biologic effectiveness (RBE) is the relative capability of radiations with differing linear energy transfer (LET) to produce a particular biologic reaction.

The RBE can be calculated as follows:

RBE = Dose in Gy from 250 kVp X-rays/Dose in Gy of test radiation

RBE = 25 Gy/5 Gy

RBE = 5

Remember, the RBE should not have any associated units.

3. The correct answer is (B).

The $LD_{50/30}$ for adults is estimated to be 3.0 to 4.0 Gy (300 to 400 rad). It is a measure of radiation lethality to 50 percent of the population at 30 days after the exposure. $LD_{10/20}$ (A) corresponds to lethality at 20 days. $LD_{50/60}$ (C) and $LD_{100/60}$ (D) both correspond to lethality at 60 days.

4. The correct answer is (D).

Late somatic effects of radiation may occur months to years after radiation exposure. In this case, the patient had been subjected to radiation for 25 years. The constant exposure will lead to a number of effects, including cancer, cataracts, birth defects (in subsequent generations), and life-span shortening.

Erythema is an early somatic effect of radiation. Nausea, vomiting, fatigue, epilation, and desquamation are also early somatic effects.

5. The correct answer is (B).

Permanent male sterility can result from an exposure to radiation doses of 5 Gy (500 rad) or more. It should be noted that standard radiographic examinations (such as an abdominal X-ray) will not result in such doses. A dose of 0.1 Gy (A) is synonymous with 10 rad (C)—this level of radiation exposure may depress sperm count. Radiation doses of 200 rad (D) may cause temporary sterility.

6. The correct answer is (C).

Both carcinogenesis and birth defects are stochastic effects of radiation. Cancer is a late somatic effect that may not occur until years after the initial exposure. Unfortunately, radiation-induced cancer cannot be distinguished on the basis of appearance. The most common cancers that result from radiation exposure are leukemia and thyroid malignancies. Additionally, cancer of the bone, skin, breast, lung, and liver has been linked to radiation exposure.

7. The correct answer is (B).

A cataract is an opacification of the ocular lens. Cataractogenesis is a nonstochastic effect of radiation and thus follows a linear, threshold relationship on the dose-response curve. Pathologies that correspond to the linear-quadratic, nonthreshold curve are breast cancer and leukemia. The nonlinear, threshold curve (sigmoid curve) represents a high dose response.

Following is a graphical representation of threshold and nonthreshold effects.

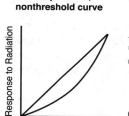

1. Linear-quadratic, nonthreshold curve

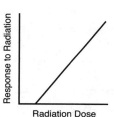

2. Linear threshold curve

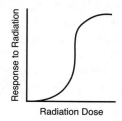

3. Nonlinear, threshold curve

8. The correct answer is (C).

The acute somatic effects of radiation occur within minutes to weeks of the time of exposure. Since the radiation worker was exposed 3 days ago, the following effects can be expected: erythema or redness of the skin (over the exposed area), epilation (loss of hair), desquamation (loss of the epidermal layer of the skin), fevers, fatigue, nausea, sterility, and hematological disorders.

The late somatic effects of radiation are observed months to years after the initial exposure. These include the stochastic effects of cancer (A) and birth defects, as well as the nonstochastic effects of cataracts (B) and life-span shortening (D).

9. The correct answer is (B).

Exposures in excess of 5,000 rad (>50 Gy) can result in a constellation of symptoms known as the central nervous system syndrome. The symptoms include anxiety, disorientation, coma, and seizures. Death often rapidly ensues. The cause of death is related to meningitis, vasculitis, or raised intracranial pressure (ICP). The cardiovascular syndrome (A) and hepatic syndrome (C) are not results of radiation exposure. The hematologic syndrome (C) occurs in response to doses between 200 and 1,000 rad. It affects the blood and blood-forming organs.

10. The correct answer is (B).

Of the different hematologic cells, lymphocytes or white blood cells are the first to become affected by radiation. Thrombocytes (platelets) and erythrocytes (red blood cells) may also be damaged. Astrocytes (A) and oligodendrocytes (D) are cells of the central nervous system. Damage to these cells would not result not result in hematologic abnormalities. Myocytes (C) are cardiac cells.

11. The correct answer is (D).

The biologic response of skin to radiation is a result of damage to the basal layer of the epidermis. A variety of conditions can result from radiation-induced skin damage. Erythema is a reddening of the skin that occurs in response to doses of 3 Gy or more. Desquamation (sloughing of the skin) often follows erythema. Epilation or loss of hair is also a response of the skin to radiation.

12. The correct answer is (B).

The gastrointestinal syndrome is a constellation of the following symptoms: anorexia, diarrhea, nausea, and vomiting. Severe diarrhea can lead to dehydration, electrolyte imbalance, and even death. The GI syndrome occurs acutely following exposure to a dose of 1,000 to 5,000 rad. Radiation doses in excess of 5,000 rad can result in ataxia (loss of balance), headaches, anxiety, disorientation, seizures, coma, and eventually death. Collectively, these symptoms are referred to as the central nervous system syndrome (A). The ensuing cause of death is often meningitis or raised intracranial pressure (ICP). Hematologic cells (white blood cells, platelets, and red blood cells) are adversely affected with the exposure to doses between 200 and 1,000 rad. The hematologic syndrome (C) is evidenced clinically by a decreased number of lymphocytes, platelets, and erythrocytes. The renal syndrome (D) is not a known response to radiation.

13. The correct answer is (B).

Organogenesis (organ development) occurs from the gestational period of 10 days to 6 weeks. Abnormalities that can occur at this stage include mental retardation, microcephaly, genital deformities, and ocular malformations.

14. The correct answer is (C).

The genetically significant dose (GSD) extrapolates the effect of gonadal radiation as if it were to be evenly distributed across the entire population. Subsequently, the consequences of gonadal radiation are reduced when averaged across the population. Bone-marrow dose (A) simply refers to the average radiation dose received by the hematopoically active cells of the bone marrow. Entrance skin exposure, or ESE (B), can be measured with a thermoluminescent dosimeter (TLD). Generally, PA films will have a lower ESE. Relative biologic effectiveness (D) is a measurement that determines whether the type of radiation used will cause biological damage.

15. The correct answer is (D).

The four types of gonadal shielding are: clear lead, flat contact, shadow shields, and shaped contact shields. Gonadal shielding is a secondary protective measure. However, adequate collimation is of primary importance. Some form of gonadal shielding device should be utilized if the patient's reproductive organs are within 5 cm of the primary beam.

16. The correct answer is (A).

Lines A and B represent a linear, nonthreshold relationship. Since both lines intersect the x-axis (dose) at zero, neither has a dose threshold. Similarly, lines C and D intersect the x-axis at points that are greater than zero. In other words, these lines are linear, threshold. Remember, the intersection of the line with the x-axis (representing dose) determines whether or not there is a threshold.

17. The correct answer is (C).

The law of Bergonie and Tribondeau states that cellular radiosensitivity can be correlated to the metabolic state of the irradiated tissue. Cells that are the least mature, such as stem cells or pleuripotent cells, are the most sensitive to the effects of radiation. Similarly, highly metabolically active cells are radiosensitive. The oxygen enhancement ratio (OER) describes the ratio of the radiation dose that results in a biologic response (A). In fact, most cells are likely to undergo programmed cell death (B) or apoptosis; however, this was not described by Bergonie and Tribondeau. The stochastic effects of radiation (D) include carcinogenesis and life-span shortening.

18. The correct answer is (A).

Programmed cell death or apoptosis is a natural process. However, it can also occur in response to radiation. Direct action (B) of ionizing radiation with RNA, DNA, enzymes, or proteins may lead to cellular damage. It is a result of interaction with high LET radiation. A point mutation (C) is damage to the structure of DNA. Often it is a result of low LET radiation. A single strand break (D) involves damage to the nitrogenous bases of DNA. Typically, it is a response to low LET.

19. The correct answer is (B).

Increased linear energy transfer (LET) results in increased radiosensitivity. Furthermore, the presence of oxygen enhances the effects of radiation on the cell. Immature cells that are exposed to high LET and increased oxygen concentrations are most radiosensitive. Anoxia (A) is the absence of oxygen, whereas hypoxia (C) is a low level of oxygenation-and neither would promote radiosensitivity.

20. The correct answer is (B).

When ionizing radiation interacts with the water molecule it produces free radicals and ions. The free radicals form hydrogen peroxide and hydroperoxyl radicals that are toxic to the cell. Most interactions with ionizing radiation result from indirect action.

21. The correct answer is (D).

The S or synthesis phase may last for up to 15 hours. During this time, DNA is synthesized. G_1 (A) is the pre-DNA synthesis phase in which RNA is produced. Proteins and RNA are assembled throughout the G_2 (B) phase. Mitosis is initiated after this phase. Prophase (C) is a component of mitosis or cell division. The other stages of mitosis are metaphase, anaphase, and telophase.

22. The correct answer is (B).

The linear-quadratic, nonthreshold curve estimates the risk associated with low LET radiation. Radiation-induced leukemia and breast cancer are represented by this curve. The linear, nonthreshold curve (A) represents the biologic response to most cancers. The sigmoid, threshold curve (C) is utilized to demonstrate a high-dose cellular response. The linear, threshold curve (D) represents the nonstochastic effects of radiation.

23. The correct answer is (C).

Linear energy transfer (LET), the oxygen enhancement ratio (OER), and the relative biologic effectiveness (RBE) are three important concepts that must be studied to understand radiation effects in tissue. LET is the average energy deposited along the path of the X-ray. The OER is the ratio of radiation dose required to cause a biologic response with and without oxygen. The RBE defines whether radiation with differing LETs will cause biologic damage. According to the Target theory, cell death ensues if the most integral component of the cell (DNA) is damaged by ionizing radiation.

24. The correct answer is (D).

If the principle of genetically significant dose (GSD) is applied to this scenario, the genetic effect observed in Group A is identical to that of Group B. Therefore, if the dose is distributed over a large population, the GSD decreases.

25. The correct answer is (C).

Following a dose of ionizing radiation, oxygenated cells have the highest rate of recovery. These cells receive more nutrients. Oxygen is a necessary component of cellular metabolism. Therefore, hypoxic and deoxygenated cells have a low rate of recovery.

26. The correct answer is (D).

Ionizing radiation causes a tremendous amount of biologic damage to humans. All of the aforementioned factors determine the level of somatic and genetic damage that result from exposure to ionizing radiation. Another factor is the ability of radiation to ionize human tissue.

27. The correct answer is (A).

High LET radiation includes particles that possess a large mass and charge because these particles deposit more energy into a small area. Such particles are more destructive to biologic matter than low LET radiation. Examples of low LET radiation are gamma rays (C) and X-rays (D).

28. The correct answer is (D).

A significant portion of the human body consists of water. Ionizing radiation interacts with the water molecule to form free radicals. These free radicals then damage cellular structures—this is an indirect effect of radiation.

Minimizing Patient Exposure

1. The correct answer is (D).

Use of intermittent fluoroscopy reduces the amount of patient dose and tube longevity. This is vital during lengthy examinations such as stent placement, filter replacement, and biliary drainage.

2. The correct answer is (A).

The air-gap technique is an alternative method that is used when a radiographic grid is not available. The air gap reduces patient dose by decreasing scatter radiation. This is achieved by increasing source-to-image distance (SID). In the trauma setting, both an AP (C) and lateral view of the cervical spine should be obtained—one should not be taken in the place of the other. During a trauma procedure, the patient should not be made to stand for a lateral cervical spine film (D).

3. The correct answer is (B).

Even though both provide an adequate diagnostic image, Figure B is an example of a low-energy X-ray beam that results in a high patient dose. In contrast, Figure A is an example of a high-energy penetrating beam. Such a beam would considerably reduce patient dose.

4. The correct answer is (B).

Using a higher film-screen exposure reduces patient exposure by about 50 percent. When the amount of silver halide crystals increases, the speed of the film is increased. Thus, a lower exposure rate is required to attain an image, which results in a lower patient dose.

5. The correct answer is (D).

In a departmental setting, repeat analysis programs are beneficial. They increase staff awareness and allow for the production of optimal films. An in-service review program will reduce film volume and repeat radiographs. This is achieved by reviewing films with the staff and identifying areas of weakness.

6. The correct answer is (B).

All of the choices are used to determine patient exposure, but entrance skin exposure (ESE) is the simplest to ascertain. A thermoluminescent dosimeter (TLD) is used to determine entrance skin dose. Because the TLD reacts to radiation in the same way that human tissue does, an accurate reading can be made.

7. The correct answer is (D).

In an extreme situation such as the one described here, it is necessary to use every possible measure to protect both the mother and fetus. Before acquiring any radiographic images the physician should conduct a thorough assessment of the patient. The radiographs should be taken only if absolutely necessary to rule out fracture.

8. The correct answer is (D).

Lengthy radiographic examinations, such as the small bowel series, result in a high patient dose.

9. The correct answer is (C).

The heartbeat is an example of involuntary motion. It is important for the radiographer to know the difference between voluntary and involuntary motion. Motion can be reduced by using shorter exposure times, high mA, and high-speed image receptors. Breathing (A), coughing (B), and laughing (D) are examples of voluntary motion.

10. The correct answer is (A).

When pathology is considered to be destructive it causes the tissue to be more radiolucent. Radiolucent tissue attenuates less X-rays and appears black on the radiograph. Patients with emphysema require reduced technique due to the presence of radiolucent tissue. Examples of radiolucent pathology are active tuberculosis, cancer, and osteoporosis. On the contrary, radiopaque pathology includes ascites, cirrhosis, pneumonia, and pleural effusion.

11. The correct answer is (B).

The relationship between time and exposure rate is directly proportional. Reducing the time by half will reduce the exposure rate by 50 percent.

Use the following to solve the problem.

$$\frac{12 \text{ mrem}}{1 \text{ second}} = \frac{x}{0.5 \text{ seconds}}$$

$$x = 6 \text{ mrem}$$

12. The correct answer is (B).

A collimator is a device that can be used to pinpoint the area of interest during an exposure. This reduces patient dose considerably. The Bucky tray (A) is part of the X-ray unit and should be used to image thicker body parts. It is not used in controlling the size of the X-ray field. The Geiger-Müller detector (C) is used as a radiation monitoring device. It has no effect on the size of the X-ray field. A grid (D) is also helpful in reducing patient dose, but it cannot control the size of the X-ray field.

13. The correct answer is (A).

It is important to remember that the entrance dose is always greater than the exit dose during radiographic procedures. Therefore, performing the abdominal radiograph in a PA projection will reduce gonadal dose. OID (B), radiographic contrast (C), and technique (D) are not affected.

14. The correct answer is (B).

Compared to cassettes that do not have screens, those with intensifying screens can reduce patient dose by about 95 percent. Film speed is relative to the amount of silver halide crystals (C) contained in the emulsion (A) of the X-ray film (D). Therefore, lower technique is required and patient dose is reduced.

15. The correct answer is (D).

Mislabeling or forgetting to indicate the anatomic site of interest can result in a repeat radiograph. Unnecessary examinations, such as repeat radiographs, can increase patient dose. Therefore, carelessness on the part of the radiographer can increase patient exposure.

16. The correct answer is (C).

The image intensification system increases image brightness. This allows the physician to use core vision. In addition, the exposure is decreased; this, in turn, reduces patient dose. Remember, improved visualization of smaller objects is an advantage of high-level control fluoroscopy.

17. The correct answer is (B).

The cone, aperture diaphragm, and collimator are examples of beam limitation devices; the most commonly used is the collimator. These devices decrease patient dose and increase image quality by limiting the beam to the area of interest. Cones are attached to the X-ray tube housing. There are two types of cones: cylindrical and flared.

18. The correct answer is (C).

Filtration reduces the amount of skin dose by absorbing low-energy photons. Appropriate filtration must be provided on X-ray units depending upon the kilovoltage (kVp). Any X-ray unit that operates above 70 kVp requires total filtration of 2.5 mm/Al. Similarly, any X-ray unit that operates within the range of 50 to 70 kVp requires total filtration of 1.5 mm/Al (A). Filtration of 2.3 mm/Al (B) is the required minimum half-value layer (HVL) for an X-ray unit operating at 80 kVp. Finally, 3.0 mm/Al (D) is the minimum half-value layer (HVL) required with units that operate at 110 kVp.

19. The correct answer is (D).

Flat contact shields are most effective when the patient is in an AP or PA recumbent position. If a flat contact shield is being used during a fluoroscopic examination, it should be placed under the patient because the X-ray tube is located under the radiographic table.

20. The correct answer is (A).

Clear lead shields should be provided for patients who receive a scoliosis exam. This allows the radiographer to visually minimize the area that needs to be irradiated. Shaped contact shields can be placed directly on the patient and are often used to shield male reproductive organs. Shadow shields are suspended from the X-ray tube itself. These protective devices can also be used to protect the gonads from the harmful effects of ionizing radiation.

21. The correct answer is (C).

Compensating filters attenuate X-rays directed toward the thinner parts of the body while allowing thicker parts of the body to receive radiation. This reduces exposure to the less dense areas of the body. The wedge filter is an example of a compensating filter that is utilized while attaining an AP projection of the foot. The aperture diaphragm (A) and the collimator (B) are examples of beam limitation devices. The lead shield (D) is a secondary protective device that minimizes patient exposure.

22. The correct answer is (D).

In selecting appropriate technical factors, the film-screen combination, quantity of filtration of the radiographic unit, and the source-to-image distance (SID) should be considered. Other factors that can also aid in the selection of technical factors include the radiographic density and contrast, and the type of X-ray generator.

23. The correct answer is (B).

A grid is used to clean up scatter before it reaches the film. The grid material, which usually consists of lead, absorbs scatter radiation. Meanwhile, the interspace material consists of aluminum or plastic that allows the X-rays to pass through. This technique reduces scatter, thus reducing patient dose.

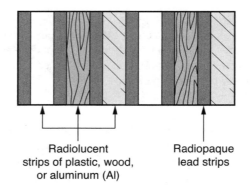

Radiolucent
strips of plastic, wood,
or aluminum (Al)

Radiopaque
lead strips

24. The correct answer is (C).   15″

With fluoroscopic procedures, the source-to-skin distance should not be less than 38 cm on stationary units. Increasing SID effectively decreases patient dose. Mobile fluoroscopic units should not have an SID of less than 30 cm (B).

                                        12″

25. The correct answer is (B).

Unnecessary radiographs can be eliminated by the proper evaluation of a patient's history by a physician. Although not all hospital admissions warrant a radiographic evaluation, patients admitted with cardiovascular or pulmonary pathology should receive a chest X-ray. Ultimately, the physician should determine which studies are necessary. Chest X-rays should not be used as a routine evaluation in a pre-employment physical. Generally, radiographs should not be obtained for patients who present without any obvious pathology. Furthermore, the chest X-ray should not be used to screen patients for tuberculosis.

26. The correct answer is (B).

Even though all of the aforementioned modalities increase occupational exposure, general fluoroscopy imaging results in the highest occupational exposure. During fluoroscopic exams, the radiographer should stand as far away from the patient as possible. While assisting the physician, the technologist should wear a lead apron and a thyroid shield.

27. The correct answer is (B).

The cumulative timer uses an audible signal to indicate that 5 minutes of fluoroscopic exposure has occurred. Effectively, this will make health care personnel more aware of radiation exposure.

28. The correct answer is (D).

Proper care of the patient in an imaging facility begins with effective communication. It is the primary responsibility of the radiographer to communicate the details of the exam to the patient. This should reduce patient anxiety and resultant uncooperative behavior. As such, repeat radiographs can be decreased considerably.

29. The correct answer is (D).

Filtration removes low-energy photons from the heterogeneous beam. This increases beam quality ("hardens" the beam) and reduces exposure to the patient's skin. Since the beam is more penetrating, it is less likely to be absorbed by superficial tissue.

30. The correct answer is (D).

The aperture diaphragm, cone, collimator, and cylinder are examples of beam limitation devices. These devices are utilized to restrict the primary or useful beam to the area of clinical interest. In doing so, the radiographer can prevent unnecessary exposure, reduce scatter, and reduce the amount of absorbed radiation.

31. The correct answer is (A).

Automatic exposure control (AEC) is a feature of the radiographic unit that measures the quantity of radiation that reaches the image receptor. This feature automatically terminates once a sufficient amount of X-rays have reached the image receptor. Lateral cells were chosen for this particular exam because a pleural effusion was being evaluated. Furthermore, a density of +1 was set to increase the optical density of the film to account for the effusion. Even though this is an automatic exposure system, the radiographer still must select the appropriate technique.

32. The correct answer is (D).

The use of a higher grid ratio will require a higher mAs. Unfortunately, this will increase patient dose. A 6:1 ratio grid (A) will require a considerably lower mAs than using a 16:1 ratio (D).

Personnel Protection

1. The correct answer is (D).

The lead apron and gloves should be imaged for cracks and leaks on a yearly basis. To prevent cracking, the protective apparel should be hung up. Thus, the lead apron will be flat. However, if the protective apparel does not meet federal standards, it should be replaced.

2. The correct answer is (D).

Time, distance, and shielding are the three basic methods of protection. Decreasing exposure time will reduce dose. Increasing distance will decrease dose. An increase in shielding will result in a decrease in dose.

3. The correct answer is (C).

The secondary protective barrier is located parallel to the X-ray beam; it shields against secondary radiation. The primary protective barrier is located perpendicular to the X-ray beam; it protects both personnel and patients from the primary beam. The control booth barrier is part of the radiographic equipment; this serves as a secondary protective barrier.

4. The correct answer is (D).

Rotating personnel through several modalities will decrease exposure by reducing the amount of time spent in areas of high exposure. When time spent in high-radiation areas is reduced, personnel exposure is also reduced. An example of such a modality is diagnostic fluoroscopy. Although providing an additional dosimeter to all personnel (A) and keeping detailed records of number of examinations performed (B) are both components of adequate monitoring, neither will reduce exposure. Finally, providing employees with one day off during the week (C) is not a practical method of reducing exposure.

5. The correct answer is (A).

Due to the increase in part thickness, the abdominal X-ray will cause more scatter. X-rays of the forearm (B) and pelvis (C) will be more defined as a result of the bony structures. Therefore, the amount of scatter radiation is less compared to the abdominal film. Incidentally, scatter can be reduced in this abdominal X-ray by using proper exposure techniques and an adequate radiographic grid.

6. The correct answer is (A).

According to the inverse square law, as the distance increases the intensity decreases by the square of its distance. So in this example, doubling the distance will decrease the intensity by a factor of 4.

Distance	Intensity
2 × distance	1/4 intensity
3 × distance	1/9 intensity

7. The correct answer is (B).

The image intensifier side (patient side) is the location that has the least amount of scatter. Since the surgeon is working in a sterile area, it would not be advisable to stand behind her (A). The radiographer should not be near the X-ray side (C); this would place him near the primary beam. The technologist cannot properly operate the C-arm from outside the operating room (D).

8. The correct answer is (D).

There are a number of considerations before designing a radiation barrier for an X-ray room. The thickness of the barrier must be increased if the occupancy factor, use factor, or workload is increased. The occupancy factor considers the use of the space adjacent to the room. The use factor is the time that the location will be exposed to the useful beam. Finally, the workload is the number of radiographic procedures performed on a weekly basis.

9. The correct answer is (B).

Leakage radiation is generated in the X-ray tube. This radiation "leaks" through the protective tube housing and is always present when the X-ray tube is on. Both leakage and scatter radiation (D) are known as secondary radiation. Primary radiation (C) comes directly from the X-ray tube and is considered to be the most damaging of all three. The technologist should avoid proximity to the primary beam.

10. The correct answer is (C).

The patient is responsible for most of the scatter radiation produced. Compton scatter is the primary interaction produced when X-rays encounter the object. This form of secondary radiation is isotropic; this causes small-angle scatter, back scatter, and side scatter. Thus, Compton scatter increases personnel exposure.

11. The correct answer is (A).

Protective curtains are placed between the clinician and the patient to reduce personnel exposure. According to the standard, the minimum lead equivalent is 0.25 mm Pb. For protective eyeglasses, 0.35 mm Pb (B) is the minimum lead equivalent. For thyroid shields, 0.50 mm Pb (C) is the minimum lead equivalent.

12. The correct answer is (B).

Increasing distance will reduce exposure. This is evidenced by the inverse square law. Reducing the distance between the primary beam and the radiographer is of paramount importance. Most scatter is produced by the patient. Thus, distance is an effective means of avoiding scatter radiation. Shielding is another effective way to decrease both patient and personnel exposure. Appropriate technique selection (i.e., exposure rate) should influence the image quality of a radiograph and reduce patient dose.

13. The correct answer is (C).

The standard exposure rate limit for a general fluoroscopic unit is 10 R/min. Nonintensified fluoroscopic units cannot exceed an exposure rate of 5 R/min (A). It should be noted that an exposure rate of 5 R/min and $5 \times 2.58 \times 10^{-4}$ C/kg/min (B) are synonymous. Units designed for high-level control (HLC) may permit exposure rates of 20 R/min (D). Since fluoroscopic examinations lead to increased patient dose, exposure rates must be kept well below established limits.

14. The correct answer is (A).

The cumulative timer should be utilized during fluoroscopic examinations. The audible signal alerts the physician after 5 minutes of fluoro time. This device is used to reduce both personnel and patient exposure. The electronic timer (B) is the most sophisticated and accurate of all the timers. It can be used for rapid serial exposures and allow for a wide range of time intervals. The exposure timer (C) can cause the X-ray tube to emit radiation for a specific amount of time predetermined by the radiographer. The mAs timer (D) is a product of milliamperage (mA) and time (sec). This timer terminates the exposure once the desired mAs has been achieved.

15. The correct answer is (D).

The Bucky slot cover attenuates scatter radiation. It must have a minimum lead equivalent of 0.25 mm Pb. Due to its placement, the Bucky slot cover is useful in the reduction of gonadal dose. A protective lead apron and lead gloves also have minimum lead equivalents of 0.25 mm Pb. If the protective curtain and the Bucky slot cover are not used simultaneously, the exposure rate to personnel would exceed 100 mR/hour at a distance of 2 feet.

16. The correct answer is (D).

Gonadal shielding should be provided for all radiographic examinations. However, in this example, placing gonadal shields on a patient receiving a KUB (C), AP pelvis (A), or AP sacrum-coccyx (B) will obscure the area of interest.

17. The correct answer is (C).

To reduce the mother's exposure she should be placed as far as possible from the primary beam. In this instance, the appropriate placement should be on the left side of the patient, thus reducing exposure to her eyes, thyroid, and breasts.

The mother is most likely to receive more exposure on the patient's right side (D) because the primary beam is directed onto the right hip.

Positioning the mother at the end or head of the table (A and B) would reduce exposure; however, she would be ineffective in the attempt to immobilize the patient.

18. The correct answer is (B).

Shielding from the primary radiation source considerably reduces occupational exposure. The door of the X-ray suite and the lead walls are examples of primary barriers. The control booth (A), the lead apron (C), and the walls of the X-ray suite that are more than 7 feet high (D) are examples of secondary barriers.

19. The correct answer is (B).

Compton scatter occurs when photons from the X-ray beam dislodge electrons. These photons then scatter in different directions (angle, back, side). Coherent scatter is also known as unmodified scatter. In this case, the photons from the X-ray beams set bound electrons into motion. The photoelectric effect involves low-energy photons and is related to patient dose.

20. The correct answer is (D).

The protective curtain should be placed between the patient and the clinician and should have a lead equivalent of 0.25 mm. The cumulative timer is a feature of the fluoroscopic tube that alerts the radiologist when the exposure time has exceeded 5 minutes. The exposure switch is a foot pedal designed to terminate exposure in case the operator becomes incapacitated. It should be a dead-man type.

Radiation Exposure and Monitoring

1. The correct answer is (A).

Extremity dosimeters should be provided to radiologists as a secondary badge. These are used to measure the amount of exposure received by the extremities while near the primary beam. Film badges (B) and thermoluminescent dosimeters (D) are personal dosimeters that are worn on the trunk. Lead gloves (C) are protective apparel that can be used during a procedure.

2. The correct answer is (B).

The Cumulative Occupational dose limit for radiation personnel is 10 mSv/year x age in years. Even though exposure limits are provided, it is still the responsibility of the radiographer to maintain a record of his or her dose limit.

3. The correct answer is (C).

Radiation equivalent man (rem) quantifies dose equivalent. The rem may be obtained by calculating the product of the absorbed dose (rad) and the quality factor (QF).

4. The correct answer is (C).

It is the responsibility of the imaging facility to keep updated personnel monitoring reports. Monthly dose-equivalent data, including deep, eye, and shallow radiation exposure, should be included. The report should also contain the type of dosimeter that was utilized. This serves as an indication of the particular modality involved.

5. The correct answer is (C).

The pocket dosimeter is the most sensitive personnel dosimeter. It contains both a positive and a negatively charged electrode. These two electrodes are exposed to ionizing radiation and indicate the level of exposure. However, these dosimeters are expensive and least frequently used. It should be noted that none of the other personnel dosimeters resembles a fountain pen.

6. The correct answer is (A).

The annual effective dose limit for members of the general public general population is 5 mSv (0.5 mrem). The annual occupational effective dose for health care workers is 50 mSv (5 mrem).

7. The correct answer is (C).

Radiation survey instruments for area monitoring are required to meet certain standards. These devices must be easy to carry, durable, and cost-effective, and designed for single-person operation. Finally, they should detect all common types of radiation. The dosimeter measures the cumulative radiation intensity.

8. The correct answer is (B).

The annual effective dose limit for clinical students is 0.1 rem, or 1 mSv. The monthly equivalent dose for the embryo-fetus is 0.05 rem (A), or 0.5 mSv. For the lens of the eye for those who receive educational exposure, the limit is 1.5 rem (C), or 15 mSv. For the skin, hands, and feet of the general population, 5 rem (D), or 50mSv, is the dose limit. This latter value is also applicable for those who receive an educational exposure.

9. The correct answer is (D).

Pregnant staff can continue to perform radiologic procedures if radiation safety measures provided by the imaging facility are adhered to. This ensures the safety of both the radiographer and the fetus. Once the pregnancy has been declared, the radiographer should be counseled by the radiation safety officer. An additional dosimeter should also be provided. This second dosimeter is given to ensure that the monthly equivalent dose to the embryo-fetus does not exceed 0.5 mSv (0.05 rem). Finally, a monthly report detailing exposure to both the radiographer and the embryo-fetus should be sent to the radiation safety officer.

10. The correct answer is (D).

To find the Cumulative Occupational dose, use the following formula:

Cumulative Occupational Dose = 10 mSv/year × age in years

Cumulative Occupational Dose = 10 mSv/year × 27

Cumulative Occupational Dose = 270 mSv

The cumulative dose equivalent should be reported for a period of 3 months.

KAPLAN

11. The correct answer is (B).

Roentgen is a measure of exposure to X-rays and gamma radiation. It is used to measure energies only up to 3 MeV. The product of absorbed dose and the quality factor will yield the rem. In addition, the product of the rad and quality factor will also yield the same result. Both equations are mathematical representations of radiation equivalent man.

12. The correct answer is (B).

When radiation interacts with an object, it deposits energy, and the rad can be applied to any type of radiation. Gray is the SI unit of radiation absorbed dose. The Coulomb per kilogram (A) is the SI unit for Roentgen. Roentgen (C) provides a measure of exposure to X-rays and gamma radiation, but it is not an SI unit. Sievert (D) is the SI unit for radiation equivalent man (rem).

13. The correct answer is (C).

Even though pocket dosimeters provide immediate exposure readings, these devices are not frequently used in diagnostic facilities. Such dosimeters are often used to monitor nonimaging personnel (e.g., nursing staff, medical students). Pocket dosimeters resemble fountain pens.

14. The correct answer is (A).

The dose equivalent summarizes aspects of different ionizing radiation that may cause biologic harm. Linear energy transfer (B) is the average energy that is deposited by ionizing radiation as it travels. The occupancy factor (C) is used to describe the utilization of the space adjacent to the X-ray source. Radiation absorbed dose (D) represents the energy that radiation transfers to an object.

15. The correct answer is (B).

A personal dosimeter can be used to assess the working habits of the technologist. Furthermore, it is indicative of the working conditions of the facility. In other words, such devices ensure that personnel are not being exposed to radiation due to inadequate shielding, faulty machines, or other structural deficits. However, personal dosimeters do not indicate the total number of exams that have been performed.

16. The correct answer is (B).

This instrument can detect the presence of electrons that have been emitted by radioactive particles. An audible alert will sound that indicates the presence of radiation. The ionization chamber-type survey meter (C) detects the presence of gamma and beta radiation. The proportional counter (D) is not used in diagnostic imaging.

17. The correct answer is (D).

Shielding is one of the primary methods of protection from ionizing radiation. General fluoroscopy results in the highest amount of personnel exposure. To ensure safety, protective apparel must be worn during the examination. The lead apron provides shielding to the trunk of the body, whereas the thyroid shield provides shielding for this sensitive endocrine organ. An extremity dosimeter is provided to the physician when her hands are required to be near the primary beam. This device will measure the dose equivalent for the hands.

18. The correct answer is (D).

Proportional counters are generally used in laboratories to detect alpha radiation, beta radiation, and low-level radioactive contamination. The Geiger-Müller (G-M) detector (A) monitors an area that has been contaminated with radioactive material. The ionization chamber-type survey meter (B) is used to measure exposure rates to both gamma rays and X-rays. An optically stimulated luminescence dosimeter (C) can be used for monitoring both workers who are employed in low-radiation environments and pregnant workers.

19. The correct answer is (D).

The radiographer should strive to keep exposure as low as reasonably achievable (ALARA). The three cardinal principles of radiation protection are time, distance, and shielding. Both distance and shielding should be maximized, while the amount of time that the patient is exposed to radiation should be kept to a minimum.

20. The correct answer is (D).

The thermal luminescent dosimeter (TLD) can be used to determine entrance skin exposure (ESE). This dosimeter has a number of advantages, including the fact that it is not affected by humidity, pressure, or temperature changes. Furthermore, LiF crystals can be reused following each reading. The TLD is the most accurate of all dosimeters—it can be worn for up to 3 months.

Chapter 8: Equipment Operation and Quality Control

Principles of Radiation Physics

1. The cloud of electrons surrounding the cathode during X-ray production is produced by which process?

   (A) Thermostatic electrification

   (B) Thermionic electrification

   (C) Thermostatic emission

   (D) Thermionic emission

2. During X-ray production, electrons travel from

   (A) anode to cathode at the speed of light.

   (B) anode to cathode at half the speed of light.

   (C) cathode to anode at half the speed of light.

   (D) cathode to anode at the speed of light.

3. The purpose of the negatively charged focusing cup that surrounds the cathode filament is to

   (A) remove electrons from the cathode filament.

   (B) reduce the size of the electron stream.

   (C) protect the cathode from incident electrons.

   (D) divert heat from the cathode filament.

4. Approximately what percentage of incident electron interactions leads to the production of X-rays?

   (A) 1%

   (B) 15%

   (C) 85%

   (D) 99%

5. X-rays produced by the slowing down or stopping of an incident electron due to the effects of the target material's nuclear force field are said to be created by what type of interaction?

   (A) Bremsstrahlung

   (B) Characteristic

   (C) Compton

   (D) Coherent

Quantum Number	Binding Energy (kEv)
1	50
2	30
3	10
4	5

6. The table above lists the binding energies for each quantum number of a made-up atom. If this atom was used as a target material, which of the following kEv levels would be a possibility for an X-ray photon created through a characteristic interaction?

   1. 5 kEv
   2. 15 kEv
   3. 20 kEv

   (A) 1 and 2 only

   (B) 1 and 3 only

   (C) 2 and 3 only

   (D) 1, 2, and 3

7. A high-energy X-ray can be described as having a

(A) short wavelength and high frequency.

(B) short wavelength and low frequency.

(C) long wavelength and low frequency.

(D) long wavelength and high frequency.

8. The quality of an X-ray beam is controlled by

(A) kVp and is primarily responsible for the number of X-rays produced.

(B) mAs and is primarily responsible for the energy of the X-rays produced.

(C) mAs and is primarily responsible for the number of X-rays produced.

(D) kVp and is primarily responsible for the energy of the X-rays produced.

9. In order to increase the number of electrons that strike the target without changing the average energy of the X-ray beam, which of the following factors can be increased?

1. kVp
2. mA
3. Time

(A) 1 and 2 only

(B) 1 and 3 only

(C) 2 and 3 only

(D) 1, 2, and 3

10. The portion of the X-ray beam that travels through the patient and produces the latent image on the image receptor is known as

(A) primary radiation.

(B) scatter radiation.

(C) remnant radiation.

(D) attenuated radiation.

11. What is the primary reason why radiation intensity decreases significantly if the distance from the target area increases?

(A) Attenuation of the X-ray beam in air

(B) Divergence of the X-ray beam

(C) Weakening of X-rays over a given distance

(D) Slowing down of X-rays over a given distance

12. During a radiographic examination of a lateral knee, the X-ray beam ionizes an atom of calcium in the patient's femur. What happened to this atom due to the ionization?

(A) It has been disintegrated.

(B) It has lost an electron.

(C) It has lost a proton.

(D) It has lost a neutron.

13. What happens during the process known as the Compton effect?

(A) An outer shell electron is removed by an X-ray.

(B) An outer shell electron is removed by an electron.

(C) An inner shell electron is removed by an electron.

(D) An inner shell electron is removed by an X-ray.

14. The results of a photoelectric absorption interaction include which of the following?

1. Ejected electron
2. Scattered X-ray
3. Creation of a characteristic photon

(A) 1 and 2 only

(B) 1 and 3 only

(C) 2 and 3 only

(D) 1, 2, and 3

GO ON TO THE NEXT PAGE ⟩

KAPLAN

15. No electrons are ejected from an atom during which one of these interactions?

    (A) Compton scatter
    (B) Photoelectric absorption
    (C) Characteristic X-ray production
    (D) Coherent scatter

16. The chance that an X-ray photon will interact with tissue through a photoelectric interaction increases as the

    (A) kVp increases.
    (B) tissue's atomic number increases.
    (C) SID increases.
    (D) X-ray photon energy increases.

17. A patient with a hypersthenic body habitus will attenuate more X-rays than a patient with an asthenic body habitus because of

    (A) increased chance of photoelectric absorption.
    (B) decreased production of Compton scatter.
    (C) decreased production of coherent scatter.
    (D) increased emergence of remnant radiation.

18. What is the advantage of greatly increasing the heat in the cathode filament prior to making a radiographic exposure?

    (A) Increased photon kEv levels
    (B) Decreased stress on filament
    (C) Decreased scatter production
    (D) Increased free electron production

19. The combination of what characteristics leads to the acceleration of electrons in the X-ray tube?

    1. Long distance between anode and cathode
    2. High voltage
    3. Opposite charges between anode and cathode

    (A) 1 and 2 only
    (B) 1 and 3 only
    (C) 2 and 3 only
    (D) 1, 2, and 3

Refer to the following illustration for Question 20:

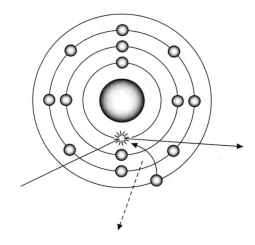

20. The X-ray illustrated in the above drawing was created through what process?

    (A) Bremsstrahlung
    (B) Compton
    (C) Pair production
    (D) Characteristic

21. The strength of an X-ray created through a bremsstrahlung interaction is determined by which of the following?

    1. The strength of the incident electron
    2. How close the incident electron passes to the nucleus
    3. The binding energies of the orbital electrons

    (A) 1 and 2 only
    (B) 1 and 3 only
    (C) 2 and 3 only
    (D) 1, 2, and 3

GO ON TO THE NEXT PAGE

KAPLAN)

Refer to the following illustration for Question 22:

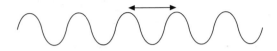

22. What electromagnetic wave characteristic is identified by the arrows in the above illustration?

    (A) Frequency
    (B) Amplitude
    (C) Wavelength
    (D) Velocity

23. The total quantity of X-rays that reach the image receptor will increase when

    (A) kVp increases or mAs increases.
    (B) kVp decreases or mAs increases.
    (C) kVp decreases or mAs decreases.
    (D) kVp increases or mAs decreases.

Refer to the following image for Question 24:

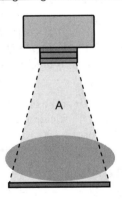

24. The portion of the X-ray beam identified by the letter A above can best be described as what portion of the X-ray beam?

    (A) Primary
    (B) Secondary
    (C) Scatter
    (D) Remnant

25. A radiographic dose of 3 mGy is measured at a distance of 80 cm from the X-ray source. If the distance is increased to 120 cm, what will be the new dose measurement?

    (A) 1.3 mGy
    (B) 2.0 mGy
    (C) 4.5 mGy
    (D) 6.8 mGy

26. Which formula determines the energy given to the photoelectron following a photoelectric absorption interaction?

    (A) Photoelectron energy = binding energy - incident photon energy
    (B) Photoelectron energy = binding energy + incident photon energy
    (C) Photoelectron energy = incident photon energy - binding energy
    (D) Photoelectron energy = incident photon energy + binding energy

27. At high kVp levels (70 kVp or above), the most common X-ray/matter interaction is

    (A) photoelectric absorption.
    (B) Compton scatter.
    (C) coherent scatter.
    (D) transmission.

28. Coherent scattering occurs only when incident photon energy

    (A) is lower than 10 kEv.
    (B) ranges from 10 to 69 kEv.
    (C) ranges from 70 to 130 kEv.
    (D) exceeds 1.2 mEv.

GO ON TO THE NEXT PAGE

29. Which one of the tissue characteristics below would produce the greatest amount of X-ray beam attenuation?

    (A) High density, high atomic number
    (B) High density, low atomic number
    (C) Low density, low atomic number
    (D) Low density, high atomic number

Radiographic Equipment

1. All operating consoles contain controls that allow for which of the following adjustments?

    1. kVp
    2. mAs
    3. SID

    (A) 1 and 2 only
    (B) 1 and 3 only
    (C) 2 and 3 only
    (D) 1, 2, and 3

2. What is the significance of using an X-ray tube that includes a dual focus arrangement?

    (A) Both kVp and mAs can be adjusted.
    (B) Both mA and time can be adjusted.
    (C) Small or large focal spot size can be selected.
    (D) Low voltage or high voltage can be selected.

3. Tungsten is an excellent metal to use as a target material for which of the following reasons?

    1. It has a high melting point.
    2. It is an excellent conductor of heat.
    3. Its atomic number leads to quality X-ray production.

    (A) 1 and 2 only
    (B) 1 and 3 only
    (C) 2 and 3 only
    (D) 1, 2, and 3

4. What is the primary job of the induction motor that is located just outside of the glass envelope of the X-ray tube?

    (A) Produce thermionic emission
    (B) Step-up voltage
    (C) Step-down voltage
    (D) Turn the rotor

5. Which list correctly describes the path of an X-ray when an ionization chamber is used to terminate the exposure?

    (A) X-ray Tube – Patient – Table – Image Receptor – Ionization Chamber
    (B) X-ray Tube – Patient – Table – Ionization Chamber – Image Receptor
    (C) X-ray Tube – Table – Patient – Ionization Chamber – Image Receptor
    (D) X-ray Tube – Ionization Chamber – Patient – Table – Image Receptor

6. In order to protect patients from excessive radiation exposure due to automatic exposure control (AEC) failure, federal law requires that when AEC is utilized during a diagnostic procedure, the generator must terminate the exposure when what mAs reading is reached?

    (A) 150 mAs
    (B) 600 mAs
    (C) 800 mAs
    (D) 1,000 mAs

7. If an exposure is made using automatic exposure control and a density control setting of -1, how will X-ray technique be affected?

    (A) kVp will be increased.
    (B) kVp will be decreased.
    (C) mAs will be increased.
    (D) mAs will be decreased.

GO ON TO THE NEXT PAGE

KAPLAN)

8. Use of a "dead-man" exposure switch ensures that

   (A) the operator cannot be exposed in the exam room.

   (B) automatic exposure controls produce the appropriate density.

   (C) an exposure cannot be made without a patient on the table.

   (D) an exposure cannot be made when the anode is stationary.

9. Positive beam limitation (PBL) devices are designed to automatically

   (A) collimate to cassette size.

   (B) center the tube to the Bucky assembly.

   (C) adjust the beam filtration.

   (D) select the correct time or mAs.

10. Which of the following requirements are necessary to create the high voltage needed for X-ray production?

    1. Alternating current
    2. Eddy currents
    3. High number of turns in the secondary coil

    (A) 1 and 2 only

    (B) 1 and 3 only

    (C) 2 and 3 only

    (D) 1, 2, and 3

Refer to the following image for Question 11:

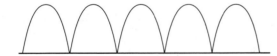

11. What is the best description of the generator waveform depicted above?

    (A) Half-wave rectified, single-phase

    (B) Full-wave rectified, single-phase

    (C) Full-wave rectified, three-phase

    (D) Half-wave rectified, three-phase

12. The input screen of a fluoroscopic unit absorbs

    (A) electrons and emits X-rays.

    (B) X-rays and emits electrons.

    (C) light photons and emits electrons.

    (D) X-rays and emits light photons.

13. What is the primary disadvantage of using a video viewing system to view a fluoroscopic image?

    (A) Image lag

    (B) Increased patient dose

    (C) Decreased resolution

    (D) Increased sensitivity

14. Which type of fluoroscopic recording device allows for repeated image transfer without quality loss?

    (A) Cine film

    (B) VHS

    (C) SVHS

    (D) Digitization

15. What is the component of a fluoroscopic unit that maintains density and contrast by manipulating mA and kVp?

    (A) Automatic gain control

    (B) Automatic brightness control

    (C) Minification control

    (D) Flux gain control

16. Which of the following events can occur inside of a photostimulable phosphor imaging plate reader?

    1. An analog signal is converted to a digital signal.
    2. Digital images are printed onto laser film.
    3. Residual information is erased from the imaging plate.

    (A) 1 and 2 only

    (B) 1 and 3 only

    (C) 2 and 3 only

    (D) 1, 2, and 3

GO ON TO THE NEXT PAGE ▷

17. Which one of the following components is responsible for collecting the latent image and sending it to a computer for processing during the creation of a direct digital radiography image?

    (A) Histogram
    (B) Photomultiplier
    (C) Spatial frequency processor
    (D) Thin film transistor

18. What is the name of the lock that secures the X-ray tube tower into place at preferred positions?

    (A) Bucky
    (B) Detent
    (C) Float switch
    (D) Collimator

19. Every mobile radiography unit must include an exposure control cord that is at least how long?

    (A) 3 feet
    (B) 6 feet
    (C) 12 feet
    (D) 15 feet

20. What is the most common target material used in a dedicated mammography unit?

    (A) Tungsten
    (B) Rhodium
    (C) Thorium
    (D) Molybdenum

21. Grid lines are often seen on a finished image when using a stationary grid. These lines will be less visible if what change is made?

    (A) Increase grid ratio
    (B) Increase grid frequency
    (C) Increase grid focus
    (D) Increase grid conversion factor

22. The Bucky assembly contains which of the following components?

    1. Movable grid
    2. Automatic exposure control detectors
    3. Cassette tray

    (A) 1 and 2 only
    (B) 1 and 3 only
    (C) 2 and 3 only
    (D) 1, 2, and 3

23. Unlike cassettes used for film-screen radiography, cassettes used for computed radiography are not designed to protect the image receptor from

    (A) rough handling.
    (B) backscatter.
    (C) blood and body fluids.
    (D) ambient light.

Refer to the following image for Question 24:

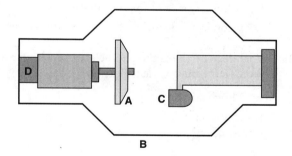

24. Which letter in the diagram above indicates the portion of the X-ray tube from which the greatest number of electrons is emitted?

    (A) A
    (B) B
    (C) C
    (D) D

GO ON TO THE NEXT PAGE

KAPLAN

25. Which one of the following generator types produces X-rays most efficiently?

    (A) High-frequency
    (B) Single-phase
    (C) Three-phase; 6-pulse
    (D) Three-phase; 12-pulse

26. What is the name given to the type of anode that does not need to be warmed up prior to making a radiographic exposure?

    (A) Rotating
    (B) Stationary
    (C) Stress-relieved
    (D) Line-focus

27. In order to protect operators from deadly electrical shock, kVp controls are located on the

    (A) primary side of the step-down transformer.
    (B) primary side of the step-up transformer.
    (C) secondary side of the step-up transformer.
    (D) secondary side of the step-down transformer.

28. What device focuses the photoelectrons within a fluoroscopic image intensification tube?

    (A) Photocathode
    (B) Input screen
    (C) Output screen
    (D) Electrostatic lens

29. Tomographic section thickness will decrease when the exposure angle

    (A) increases and the tube motion becomes more complex.
    (B) increases and the tube motion becomes less complex.
    (C) decreases and the tube motion becomes less complex.
    (D) decreases and the tube motion becomes more complex.

Quality Control of Radiography Equipment and Accessories

1. According to federal regulations, the collimated field size may not exceed the size of the collimated light field by more than

    (A) 2 percent of the SID.
    (B) 4 percent of the SID.
    (C) 4 percent of the image receptor length.
    (D) 2 percent of the image receptor length.

2. In order to ensure that the X-ray beam is centered to the image receptor, an X-ray beam Bucky tray alignment test is performed. If the SID is set to 70 cm, the test results should indicate that the center of the Bucky tray varies from the center of the X-ray field by no more than

    (A) 0.7 cm.
    (B) 1.0 cm.
    (C) 1.4 cm.
    (D) 2.0 cm.

3. A piece of radiographic equipment that has been working properly begins to produce radiographs with increased density. Several tests are performed using a technique of 400 mA, 0.20 seconds, 70 kVp, and an 80 cm SID. The results of the tests indicate that the actual readings are 400 mA, 0.21 seconds, 77 kVp, and a 79 cm SID. According to these test results, what factor is the major cause of the increased density?

    (A) SID
    (B) Time
    (C) kVp
    (D) A and C

GO ON TO THE NEXT PAGE ⟩

KAPLAN

Refer to the following radiograph for Question 4:

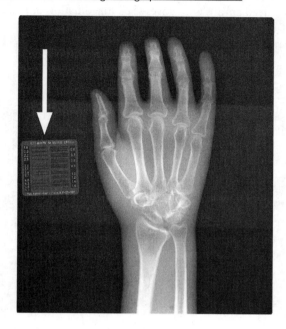

4. The tool identified by the white arrow in the image displayed above is used to measure

   (A) focal spot size.
   (B) single-phase generator time settings.
   (C) resolution.
   (D) half-value layer.

5. The focal spot size can be measured with which of the following tools?

   1. Star resolution pattern
   2. Pinhole camera
   3. Synchronous spinning top

   (A) 1 and 2 only
   (B) 1 and 3 only
   (C) 2 and 3 only
   (D) 1, 2, and 3

6. How often should lead aprons should be inspected under fluoroscopy?

   1. Upon acceptance
   2. Every 6 months
   3. Whenever a problem is suspected

   (A) 1 and 2 only
   (B) 1 and 3 only
   (C) 2 and 3 only
   (D) 1, 2, and 3

7. An image is created using a technique of 200 mA, 0.25 seconds, 75 kVp, and 100 cm SID. The mA is decreased to 100 mA and the time is increased to 0.5 seconds. The second image displays an optical density with a value 0.3 higher than the first image. This test indicates a failure of the

   (A) kVp system.
   (B) reciprocity law.
   (C) automatic exposure control.
   (D) heat sensors.

8. A light field to radiation field alignment test is performed on a 35 cm (43 cm) image receptor with an SID of 80 cm. What would be the largest acceptable variation measurement?

   (A) 0.86 cm
   (B) 1.72 cm
   (C) 3.20 cm
   (D) 1.60 cm

   $$\frac{8 \times 2}{100} = 16$$

9. What is a wire mesh test tool used to test?

   (A) Grid alignment
   (B) Half-value layer
   (C) Spatial resolution
   (D) Film-screen contact

GO ON TO THE NEXT PAGE ▷

10. If intensification screens are not cleaned regularly, what types of artifacts may begin to appear?

    (A) White specks
    (B) Black specks
    (C) Underexposed radiograph
    (D) Overexposed radiograph

11. What is the minimum acceptable thickness of the lead aprons and gloves used for radiation protection?

    (A) 0.25 mm lead-equivalent
    (B) 0.5 mm lead-equivalent
    (C) 1.0 mm lead-equivalent
    (D) 2.5 mm lead-equivalent

Answers and Explanations

Principles of Radiation Physics

1. The correct answer is (D).

An X-ray tube is constructed of two major components: a positively charged anode and a negatively charged cathode. The cathode contains a thin wire called a *filament*, through which a large number of electrons are forced during a radiographic exposure. Because large numbers of electrons are forced through such a small wire, a great deal of heat is produced and individual electrons are forced out of the wire through a process called *thermionic* (ionization due to increased heat) *emission* (forcing out). Thermostatic (A and C) refers to temperature regulation. Electrification (A and B) refers to the charging of an object generally by adding electrons, not ejecting them.

2. The correct answer is (C).

Electrons travel from the negatively charged cathode to the positively charged anode. Due to the extremely high voltage applied to the X-ray circuit, electrons from the negatively charged cathode are very quickly accelerated to nearly half the speed of light. This acceleration takes place over the very small distance of 2 cm.

3. The correct answer is (B).

Electrons carry a negative charge and will tend to move away from each other (diverge) once they have left the cathode filament. The negatively charged focusing cup prevents the electrons from straying too far away from each other by focusing the electrons into a smaller area. This is possible because like charges repel each other; therefore, the negatively charged focusing cup will repel the negatively charged electrons. The smaller electron stream results in the electrons striking a smaller area of the anode and ultimately a smaller focal spot size.

4. The correct answer is (A).

X-ray production is a very inefficient process. When incident electrons slam into the anode, heat is the most common result. Slightly more than 99 percent of the interactions caused by incident electrons lead to heat being created in the anode; therefore, slightly less than 1 percent of these interactions lead to the production of X-rays. Approximately 15 percent (B) of the interactions leading to X-ray production result in characteristic X-rays, while 85 percent (C) lead to bremsstrahlung X-ray production.

5. The correct answer is (A).

Bremsstrahlung is a German word meaning *braking* or *slowing*. As incident electrons enter the target material, they interact with the force field of the atomic nucleus, causing the electrons to slow down. When the incident electron slows down, kinetic energy is given off in the form of an X-ray. Characteristic interactions (B) are caused by the interactions of incident electrons with orbital electrons. Both Compton interactions (C) and coherent interactions (D) are the result of X-rays interacting with matter.

6. The correct answer is (B).

An X-ray created through a characteristic interaction is produced when an incident electron strikes an inner shell electron out of orbit and is replaced by an outer shell electron. The strength of the resulting X-ray is determined by the difference between the binding energies of the two orbital electrons involved. For example, if a K-shell (quantum number 1) electron is ejected and replaced by an electron from the L-shell (quantum number 2), the resulting X-ray would have a strength of 20 kEv (50 kEv - 30 kEv).

7. The correct answer is (A).

Frequency is the number of *pulses* in a wave—that is, the number of times a wave will pass a fixed point in a given period of time. Wavelength is the distance between waves. X-rays, like all other forms of electromagnetic radiation, follow the wave equation: speed = wavelength × frequency. Because all electromagnetic radiation travels at the speed of light and is therefore constant, wavelength will be decreased as frequency is increased. It is not possible, then, for electromagnetic radiation to demonstrate long wavelength and high frequency (D) or short wavelength and low frequency (B). X-rays are some of the most powerful types of electromagnetic radiation and demonstrate high frequency and low wavelength. A good rule of thumb is to equate frequency with energy; the higher the frequency, the higher the energy.

8. The correct answer is (D).

kVp controls the amount of energy given to the incident electrons that strike the target and create X-rays. When the incident electrons are given increased energy, more energy is given to the X-rays created through bremsstrahlung interactions. The amount of energy in the X-ray beam controls the quality of the beam; as energy increases, quality also increases.

9. The correct answer is (C).

Increasing the mA increases the number of electrons that are sent in the electron stream from the cathode to the anode. Increasing the time increases the amount of time that electrons are streaming from cathode to anode; this increases the total number of electrons. Increasing the kVp increases the number of X-rays that are produced but changes the average energy of the X-ray beam (quality).

10. The correct answer is (C).

The beam of X-rays that exits the X-ray tube is called *primary* radiation (A). As the X-rays pass through a patient's body, some are absorbed (attenuated; D) and some are misdirected (scattered; B). The remaining X-rays pass through the patient's body to form the latent image. The remaining radiation is called *remnant* radiation and is sometimes also referred to as *exit* radiation.

11. The correct answer is (B).

X-rays are produced *isotopically*, or in all directions from the target. The usable X-ray beam exits the X-ray tube as a cone-shaped beam with the base of the cone becoming wider as the distance from the target increases. This divergence spreads the X-rays over a wider area as they travel from the target, which reduces the intensity in a given area. X-rays are only slightly attenuated by the molecules in the air (A), and they do weaken as they travel (B). All X-rays travel at the speed of light and will not slow down (D) until they are absorbed.

12. The correct answer is (B).

Ionization is the process of removing or adding an electron to an atom. In this question the only answer that is possible is the removal of an electron from the atom, which would result in a positively charged calcium atom. This atom may remain positive for a very short period of time until a free electron fills the void created by the ionization. X-rays in the diagnostic range do not possess enough energy to remove a proton (C) or neutron (D) from the nucleus.

13. The correct answer is (A).

The Compton effect, also referred to as *Compton scatter*, occurs when an X-ray removes an outer shell electron from orbit; the X-ray then continues its journey, often in a different direction.

14. The correct answer is (B).

Photoelectric absorption occurs when an X-ray strikes an inner shell electron and removes it from orbit. During this interaction the X-ray and its energy are totally absorbed by the ejected electron; the X-ray is absorbed, not scattered. The void left by the ejected inner shell electron is filled by an outer shell electron, and a weak characteristic photon is created.

15. The correct answer is (D).

Coherent scattering occurs only when very low energy X-ray photons (10 kEv or below) interact with a single electron or all of the electrons in an atom. The energy of the incoming X-ray is absorbed, causing the electron(s) to vibrate and create a new X-ray. This new X-ray contains the same energy level as the incoming X-ray but it travels in a different direction. Because no electrons are ejected during this interaction, no ionization occurs.

16. The correct answer is (B).

The chances that an X-ray will be absorbed through the process of photoelectric absorption increases dramatically when the atomic number of the tissue or matter is increased. This is due in large part to the increased number of orbital electrons present. For example, bone has a higher average atomic number than soft tissue; more X-rays are absorbed in bone. Elements such as lead easily absorb X-rays in the diagnostic range because of its very high atomic number. When the energy of the X-ray beam is increased (A or D), the chances of a photoelectric absorption interaction actually decrease. Although increased SID (C) will lead to decreased intensity of radiation and the illusion of increased absorption, this is due to a decreased number of X-rays interacting with tissue but does not affect the interactions of a single X-ray photon.

17. The correct answer is (A).

When the thickness or density of body tissue increases, there is an increased chance of a photoelectric absorption interaction because an increased number of electrons are present and an increased chance that an X-ray will interact with one of these electrons. Of course, the increased number of atoms also leads to an increase in scatter production (B and C) and a decrease in the amount of radiation that will strike the image receptor (D) and create the latent image.

18. The correct answer is (D).

The process of thermionic emission greatly increases the heat present in the cathode filament. Heating the filament raises the energy state of orbital electrons, moving them further from the atomic nucleus and making them easier to remove. This increases the number of electrons that are available to stream from cathode to anode during the radiographic exposure. Thermionic emission does place a great deal of stress on the filament (B), however, and manufacturers have built in safeguards to protect the filament. The free electrons created through the process of thermionic emission do not directly affect scatter production (C) or the strength of resulting X-ray photons (A).

19. The correct answer is (C).

Many more electrons are present in the cathode prior to exposure, giving the cathode a negative charge when compared to the anode. These *free* electrons congregate near the cathode during the process of thermionic emission but cannot migrate to the anode due to the distance. Once the exposure button is pressed and the high voltage interacts with the free electrons near the cathode, they are quickly accelerated over the relatively short distance (2 cm) between the cathode and the anode.

20. The correct answer is (D).

X-rays produced through characteristic interactions are produced when an incident electron strikes an inner shell electron and knocks it out of orbit. To fill the void left by the ejected electron, an outer shell electron drops down to fill the void and gives off excess energy in the form of an X-ray photon. Bremsstrahlung photons are created by the interaction of an incident electron and an atomic nucleus (A). Both Compton and coherent (B and C) interactions are the result of an X-ray's interaction with orbital electrons.

21. The correct answer is (A).

Bremsstrahlung X-rays are produced when incident electrons interact with the nucleus of an atom. The closer the incident electron passes the nucleus, the more kinetic energy is given off in the form of an X-ray. An X-ray with increased kinetic energy (more energy) will have more energy available to release in the form of an X-ray. X-rays created through a bremsstrahlung interaction do not interact with orbital electrons; therefore, the binding energies of these electrons is insignificant to the strength of bremsstrahlung X-rays.

22. The correct answer is (C).

The distance between identical areas of an electromagnetic wave is called the *wavelength*. In the present case, the arrows identify the distance between the peaks of two separate waves. The height of the electromagnetic wave is called the amplitude (B). The frequency (A) of the wave is determined by how many waves pass a fixed point in a given period of time.

23. The correct answer is (A).

When mAs increases, the total number of electrons that travel from the cathode to the anode will increase; this increases the total number of X-rays created. When kVp is increased, X-ray photons more easily penetrate the tissue being exposed and reach the image receptor.

24. The correct answer is (A).

The beam of X-rays emitted from the X-ray tube is referred to as the primary beam. The primary beam has not yet undergone attenuation or scattering interactions. Secondary radiation (B) refers to the X-rays that are produced in the body as a result of photoelectric absorption. Scatter radiation

(C) refers to the portion of the primary beam that is deviated from its original path. X-rays that pass all the way through the body and form the latent image on the image receptor are referred to as remnant radiation (D).

25. The correct answer is (A).

In order to answer this question, the inverse square law must be used:

Original Intensity/New Intensity = New Distance^2/Old Distance^2

In the present case the original intensity is 3 mGy at an 80 cm SID. The new distance is 120 cm, so the problem should be set up like this:

New Intensity = $3'''\times'''80^2/120^2$

New Intensity = $3 \times 6,400/14,400$

New Intensity = 19,200/14,400

New Intensity = 1.3

26. The correct answer is (C).

During a photoelectric absorption interaction, an incident X-ray photon removes an inner shell electron from orbit. The binding energy of the orbital electron is the amount of energy needed to knock the electron out of orbit. The energy of the incident photon must by equal to or greater than the binding energy of the orbital electron in order for the orbital electron to be ejected. Because the energy of the incident photon is completely transferred during this interaction, some of the energy is used to eject the orbital electron (now called the *photoelectron*) and the remainder is given to the photoelectron in the form of kinetic energy.

27. The correct answer is (B).

The percentage of interactions that lead to Compton scatter range from 60 to 75 percent when a kVp exceeding 70 kVp is utilized. The next most common interaction is photoelectric absorption (25 to 37 percent). Coherent scatter production results in less than 1 percent of all interactions. The percentage of X-rays that do not interact with matter and are transmitted all the way through matter is dependent on tissue thickness but rarely exceeds 20 percent.

28. The correct answer is (A).

Coherent scattering is not an important factor in diagnostic imaging because it only occurs at very low energy levels. Most X-ray photons below 10 kEv have been removed from the beam as a result of beam filtration.

29. The correct answer is (A).

Tissues that contain high atomic numbers attenuate the X-ray beam more effectively because more electrons are available to interact with incident X-ray photons. Increased density also increases the number of electrons available for interaction in a given volume of tissue.

Radiographic Equipment

1. The correct answer is (A).

Adjustments to radiographic technique are made at the operating console that is always located behind a protective barrier. In addition to mAs and kVp, adjustments to time and focal spot size can also be made at the operating console. Adjustments to distance, tube angle, central ray alignment, and patient positioning are almost always made in the examination room. Some newer equipment is capable of adjusting SID, tube angle, and central ray alignment at the operating console, but this is the exception in radiographic equipment, not the rule.

2. The correct answer is (C).

When an X-ray tube uses a *dual focus* arrangement, two different filaments are built into the focusing cup. One of these filaments will produce a large stream of electrons, while the second, smaller filament will produce a smaller stream of electrons. The large and small streams of electrons correspond with the large and small focal spots created as the stream of electrons slam into the anode.

3. The correct answer is (D).

Tungsten is an excellent choice as a target material for all of the reasons listed in this question. The high melting point of tungsten (3,370ºC) means that it is capable of managing the high number of heat interactions that occur when electrons strike it. In addition, tungsten's ability to conduct heat helps to protect the anode from heat-related damage. Tungsten's atomic number, specifically its K-shell binding energy of 69.5 kEv, leads to the production of characteristic X-rays in the perfect range for diagnostic imaging.

4. The correct answer is (D).

The induction motor, or stator, is responsible for turning the rotor that turns the anode inside the X-ray tube. The spinning anode greatly reduces the ability of the anode to handle the heat created during X-ray production. The induction motor is located outside of the X-ray tube and spins the rotor through the use of a series of electromagnets.

5. The correct answer is (B).

An ionization chamber terminates an exposure when a preset amount of radiation has been detected. The ionization chamber sits between the table and the image receptor and does not normally appear on a finished image because it is very thin (approximately 5 mm). Older automatic exposure control systems known as phototimers are located behind the image receptor (A).

6. The correct answer is (B).

At kVp settings in the diagnostic range (above 50 kVp), a backup time is set to ensure that the generator does not continue to produce X-rays when a problem occurs with the AEC. This time should ideally be set at 150 percent of the anticipated time; if this does not occur, the generator must terminate the exposure when 600 mAs is reached.

7. The correct answer is (D).

Automatic exposure control (AEC) manages the time or mAs setting during a radiographic exposure; kVp must be manually set by the operator. *Density controls* allow the operator to increase or decrease the amount of radiation that must be detected by the ionization chamber in order to terminate the exposure. These controls allow the operator to compensate for anatomical or positioning variations that cannot otherwise be adjusted. A setting of -1 would decrease the mAs, while a setting of +1 would increase the mAs. Most radiographic equipment includes density controls with several steps; for example: -3, -2, -1, 0, +1, +2, +3.

8. The correct answer is (A).

A *dead-man* exposure switch ends an exposure when the switch is released. This prevents the X-ray equipment from continuing to produce radiation when the operator enters the room. It also protects the patient because the operator can release the switch and terminate the exposure prematurely if the technologist observes patient movement during the exposure.

9. The correct answer is (A).

When a cassette is placed into the Bucky assembly, the size is detected by the PBL system and the collimated area is adjusted accordingly. This ensures that the collimated area does not exceed the size of the image receptor, thereby needlessly exposing areas to radiation that will not add to the radiographic image.

10. The correct answer is (B).

In order to create voltage high enough to produce X-rays, a step-up transformer is necessary. A step-up transformer consists of two coils of wire, a primary coil (the one supplied with current) and a secondary coil (the coil in which current is induced). If the number of turns in the secondary coil exceeds the number of turns in the primary coil, voltage will be increased. If the number of turns in the secondary coil is less than the number of turns in the primary coil, voltage will be decreased (step-down transformer). All transformers need the varying magnetic field created by alternating current in order to induce voltage in a secondary coil. Eddy current refers to the current loss in a transformer as a result of conflicting forces.

11. The correct answer is (B).

Rectification refers to the changing of alternating current to pulsating direct current. This is a critical adjustment in the X-ray circuit because this type of generator waveform ensures that electrons travel only from the cathode to the anode during X-ray production. In this example, the entire waveform has been rectified so that the electrons move in pulses in the same direction rather than alternating their movement. The *phase* of the waveform refers to the number of waveforms produced by the generator. In this question, there is only one waveform so it is termed single-phase.

12. The correct answer is (D).

The image intensification tube alters energy as it travels from input screen to output screen. X-rays exit the patient and strike the input phosphor. The input phosphor immediately changes the energy from the X-rays into light photons, which are changed to electrons by the photocathode.

13. The correct answer is (C).

The limiting factor of video viewing systems is the *raster pattern* of the monitor, or the number of lines in the video image. Video viewing systems are only capable of producing resolutions of 1 to 2 lp/mm.

14. The correct answer is (D).

Storing a fluoroscopic image on Cine film or videotape may be a good short-term storage solution. However, if digital imaging is utilized and the image is digitized, an unlimited number of copies can be created without damage to the original image. In addition, the image can be sent through a PACS for remote viewing, storage, or printing.

15. The correct answer is (B).

Automatic brightness control (also known as automatic dose control or automatic brightness stabilization) automatically increases or decreases kVp and mA to compensate for changes in subject density and contrast. These adjustments maintain satisfactory density and contrast of the fluoroscopic image. Automatic gain control (A) adjusts density and contrast through the use of video adjustment but does not use changes in mA and kVp to make this alteration.

16. The correct answer is (B).

During digital imaging utilizing a computed radiography system, the latent image is captured on a photostimulable phosphor (PSP) plate. The PSP plate is fed into an analog-to-digital converter (ADC) where a laser releases the latent image in the form of light photons. The light photons are then converted to a digital image and sent to a computer for processing, or sent to a laser printer in order to print a hard-copy film.

17. The correct answer is (D).

Thin-film transistors (TFTs) are tiny components of a direct digital radiography flat-panel imaging plate. TFTs detect and capture electric charges created by the interaction of the flat-panel plate and incident X-rays. These charges are then transferred to a computer for processing by the TFTs.

18. The correct answer is (B).

Detents are preset locking positions that assist in the alignment of the tube with the image receptor, or lock in the X-ray tube tower at a desired SID. When a release button is pushed by an operator, the X-ray tube tower can be freely moved into a desired position. At specific points, the tower release will lock into position as the tube travels past a point where the tube is longitudinally or transversely centered to the image receptor.

19. The correct answer is (B).

The cord on the mobile radiographic machine ensures that the operator can stand as far as possible from the *patient*. Because scattered radiation from the patient is the primary source of radiation exposure to the radiographer, care must be taken to increase the distance from the patient with the use of the exposure control cord.

20. The correct answer is (D).

Molybdenum offers several advantages as a target material in mammography. The primary advantage of using molybdenum is that characteristic photons created in a molybdenum target contain energies in the 17 to 20 kEv range. This range of energies makes visualization of breast anatomy easier because at this energy level increased photoelectric absorption interactions occur.

21. The correct answer is (B).

Frequency refers to the number of lines per inch of lead strips that a grid contains. If the grid ratio remains constant and the frequency increases, the number of lead strips per inch will increase and the strips will become thinner and be less noticeable on the finished image. Increasing grid ratio (A) increases the thickness of the grid or the grid lines, making the grid lines even more noticeable. Increasing the grid conversion factor (D) is the same as increasing the grid ratio. Increasing the focus of the grid (C) does not affect the thickness of the lead strips.

22. The correct answer is (D).

The Bucky assembly is named after Gustav Bucky, the person who invented the radiographic grid. The Bucky assembly refers to the mechanical devices that lie between the radiographic table (or wall board) and the image receptor as well as the tray that holds the cassette in position during the exposure.

23. The correct answer is (D).

Unlike radiographic film, the phosphor plates used in computed radiography are not as sensitive to ambient room light. In fact, a phosphor plate can be removed from the cassette in normal room light and returned to the cassette prior to exposure without damage to the future latent image. The phosphor plate does, however, become slightly more sensitive to light after exposure. Although the cassette used in computed radiography does a fairly good job of keeping ambient light away from the phosphor plate, it is not considered to be as lightproof as a film-screen cassette.

24. The correct answer is (C).

The letter C in the illustration identifies the cathode. The cathode is the negatively charged side of the X-ray tube from which electrons are emitted. This emission occurs when a large cloud of electrons, separated from the cathode filament due to the effects of thermionic emission, is very quickly accelerated from the cathode to the anode by high voltage. As the electrons are quickly decelerated in the anode (A), X-rays are created and exit the tube (B).

25. The correct answer is (A).

The output of all X-ray generators fluctuates as it produces X-rays. Some generators fluctuate a great deal; for example, a single-phase unit produces X-rays and stops producing X-rays 120 times per second. The output of a single-phase unit is very inefficient due to the starting and stopping of X-ray production. High-frequency generators produce a much more constant waveform, and therefore, a much more constant production of X-rays.

26. The correct answer is (C).

When incident electrons bombard the anode, the majority of the interactions are heat interactions. Because so much heat is generated in the anode, it must be warmed up prior to use at the beginning of the day; this prevents cracking of the anode. Stress-relieved anodes are able to disperse heat much more quickly than other types of anodes and do not need to be warmed up.

27. The correct answer is (B).

The step-up transformer raises voltage from about 220 volts to more than 50,000 volts. Although receiving an electrical shock is seldom a pleasant event, an electric shock of 50,000 volts is much more dangerous than a 220-volt shock. The primary side of the step-up transformer is the side supplied with power—prior to stepping up the voltage to extremely high levels. Therefore, it is much safer to adjust the kVp on the low-voltage side of the X-ray circuit.

28. The correct answer is (D).

Photoelectrons are emitted by the photocathode inside of the image intensification tube. The fluoroscopic image is *minified* (made smaller) inside the image intensification tube as the photoelectrons travel from the photocathode to the output screen because of the actions of the electrostatic lenses. The electrostatic lenses carry a negative charge and funnel the negatively charged photoelectrons into a thinner stream as they travel. Manipulation of the electrical charge and voltage of the electrostatic lenses can affect the magnification of the fluoroscopic image as well.

29. The correct answer is (A).

The exposure angle is the distance the tomographic tube moves during the exposure. As the angle increases, the amount of blurring that occurs also increases, making a thin area of sharpness appear at the fulcrum point. The more complex the tube motion becomes, the more blurring also occurs; this also leads to a smaller section of sharpness.

Quality Control of Radiography Equipment and Accessories

1. The correct answer is (A).

When a radiographic exposure is produced, the radiation field should not extend beyond the edge of the image receptor. When this occurs, additional anatomy is exposed to radiation without contributing diagnostic information. If the resulting radiation field is smaller than the light field used for positioning, important anatomy may be omitted and the image may have to be repeated. In order to ensure that the light field used for positioning closely matches the resulting radiation field, tests are conducted to ensure that the radiation field does not vary from the light field by more than 2 percent of the SID. For example, if the SID is 100 cm, the light field and the radiation field can vary by no more than 2 cm.

2. The correct answer is (A).

The center of the Bucky tray can vary from the center of the X-ray field by no more than 1 percent of the SID. In this question the SID is 70 cm, so the variation may not exceed 1 percent of 70 cm, which is 0.7 cm.

3. The correct answer is (C).

The kVp may vary from the selected kVp by no more than 5 percent. In the present case the kVp is set to 70, so a reading greater than 5 percent, or 3.5 kVp, would indicate a problem. The kVp reading is 10 percent greater than the selected kVp, so a problem exists. The other factors are within tolerance limits (Time ± 5 percent; SID ± 2 percent).

4. The correct answer is (C).

The tool in the radiograph displayed in this image is a line pair test tool that measures resolution. Resolution is the measurement of how well small structures can be seen on a completed radiograph. Measurement is made in line pairs per millimeter (LP/mm). As the number of visible line pairs increases, the lines in the test tool become smaller and harder to discriminate from each other. Imaging systems that are able to display a higher number of line pairs are said to display increased resolution.

5. The correct answer is (A).

Both the pinhole camera and the star resolution pattern can be used to estimate the size of the true focal spot size. The synchronous spinning top is used to measure timer accuracy.

6. The correct answer is (D).

A lead apron should be inspected when it is purchased to make sure that no manufacturing defects are present. In addition, the apron should also be inspected every 6 months to ensure that cracks or shifting of the lead sheeting has not occurred. Whenever a problem is suspected with a lead apron, it should also be inspected. Problems may be suspected if cracking or shifting of the lead sheeting can be felt or seen, or if a lead apron has been folded for an extended period of time.

7. The correct answer is (B).

The reciprocity law states that a specific mAs setting should result in the same radiation output regardless of the combinations of mA and time used. In this question two mA and time settings are used to produce 50 mAs. The different mAs settings do not result in the same tube output, however, indicating a failure of the reciprocity law. Anytime the optical density of two images produced with the same mAs vary by more than 0.2, the reciprocity law is said to fail.

8. The correct answer is (D).

The collimated field size may not exceed the size of the collimated light field by more than 2 percent of the SID. In this question the SID is 80 cm, so the variation may not exceed 2 percent of 80 cm, which is 1.6 cm.

9. The correct answer is (D).

In order to test the contact of an intensification screen and radiographic film in a film-screen cassette, a wire mesh test tool is placed on the cassette and an image is produced. If an area of poor film-screen contact exists, an area of increased density and blur appears due to increased diffusion of light from the intensification screen. Cassettes with poor film-screen contact should not be used for patient examinations because spatial resolution will be decreased, important anatomy may be obscured, or the blur may imitate certain pathologies.

10. The correct answer is (A).

Dirt and dust in a radiographic cassette will eventually work their way in between the intensification screen and radiographic film. When this occurs, light from the intensification screen is not able to reach the film and a tiny area of decreased density (white speck) will occur. Dirt or dust will not affect the entire radiograph, only the area where the dust or dirt is located.

11. The correct answer is (B).

Lead aprons and gloves must provide radiation protection while still providing practicality and some degree of comfort. A lead-equivalent thickness of 0.5 mm provides radiation protection while still making an apron practical to wear for long fluoroscopic procedures.

Chapter 9: **Patient Care and Education**

Ethical and Legal Aspects

1. A radiographer who applies arm restraints to immobilize a patient without first obtaining a physician's order may be criminally charged with

   (A) false imprisonment.

   (B) assault.

   (C) battery.

   (D) negligence.

2. Radiology patient data sheets (requisitions) are legal documents and must include which of the following information?

   1. Patient name
   2. Patient history
   3. Name of radiographer performing the examination

   (A) 1 only

   (B) 1 and 2 only

   (C) 1 and 3 only

   (D) 1, 2, and 3

3. That patients are to be treated as individuals and to be informed about their procedures to facilitate appropriate decision making in their own care is the definition of

   (A) autonomy.

   (B) a living will.

   (C) a durable power of attorney.

   (D) an advance directive.

4. Informed consent will include the following elements EXCEPT which of the following?

   (A) The consent must be given voluntarily.

   (B) The consent must be in writing and signed by the patient or representative.

   (C) The consent to treat a minor should be signed by the treating physician.

   (D) The consent should include a description of the risks and benefits of the procedure, alternative treatment options, and expected outcomes.

5. If a radiographer maliciously spreads information about a patient by telling another radiographer confidential patient details, the radiographer may be guilty of

   (A) malpractice.

   (B) medical negligence.

   (C) libel.

   (D) slander.

6. If a radiographer touches a patient without justification or cause during a radiographic procedure, he or she may be legally charged with

   (A) malpractice.

   (B) negligence.

   (C) battery.

   (D) false imprisonment.

7. The radiographer's obligation to tell the truth and not lie to deceive others is called

   (A) autonomy.
   (B) veracity.
   (C) statutory disclosure.
   (D) confidentiality.

8. Which of the following are examples of an Advance Health Care Directive?

   1. Living will
   2. DNR order
   3. DNI order

   (A) 1 only
   (B) 2 only
   (C) 1 and 2 only
   (D) 1, 2, and 3

9. Which of the following terms implies that it is the radiographer's duty to maintain a professional standard of care at all times and to refrain from doing harm to a patient?

   (A) Nonmaleficence
   (B) Fidelity
   (C) Justice
   (D) Beneficence

10. The legal theory or doctrine of "Respondeat Superior" requires that the

    (A) thing speaks for itself.
    (B) employee is responsible for the employer's actions.
    (C) employee is responsible for his or her own actions.
    (D) master speaks for the servant.

11. A radiographer's breach in providing the applicable standard of care to a patient that results in harm to the patient is known as

    (A) battery.
    (B) assault.
    (C) tort.
    (D) medical malpractice.

12. The focus of HIPAA legislation mandates is that

    (A) Prospective Payment Systems (PPS) are established.
    (B) patient health information/records are held confidential.
    (C) Diagnosis-Related Group (DRG) categories are registered.
    (D) Quality management is practiced within the hospital.

13. A "No Code" order, in which a terminal patient decides no effort at resuscitation is to be attempted, is known as

    (A) DRG.
    (B) DNR.
    (C) DNI.
    (D) durable power of attorney.

14. Tort refers to

    (A) negligence.
    (B) a misdemeanor.
    (C) a felony.
    (D) a civil wrong.

GO ON TO THE NEXT PAGE

15. Which of the following are part of the Patient's Bill of Rights?

    1. The patient has the right to considerate and respectful care.
    2. The patient has the right to every consideration of privacy.
    3. The patient has the right to have an advance directive.

    (A) 1 only
    (B) 2 only
    (C) 1 and 2 only
    (D) 1, 2, and 3

Interpersonal Communication

1. According to the Kübler-Ross theory of the grieving process, the first and last steps of the five-step process that people go through as an emotional response to loss are

    (A) anger and acceptance.
    (B) denial and bargaining.
    (C) denial and acceptance.
    (D) acceptance and bargaining.

2. When recording a patient's history, an example of a subjective finding would be

    (A) an elevated BUN level.
    (B) the palpation of a lump.
    (C) the patient complaining of a sharp abdominal pain.
    (D) blood in the urine.

3. On which of the following communication skills would a blind patient rely the MOST?

    (A) Verbal
    (B) Written
    (C) Physical
    (D) Demonstration

4. The act of recognizing and entering into the feelings of another person is called

    (A) empathy.
    (B) sympathy.
    (C) similarity.
    (D) rapport.

5. What is the best method radiographers can use to control voluntary motion by the patient?

    (A) Increase the exposure time
    (B) Use immobilization devices
    (C) Communicate to the patient what will be done
    (D) Use a high kVp

6. During a radiographic examination, the radiographer should maintain eye contact with the patient. Visual contact is a form of

    (A) palpation.
    (B) examination.
    (C) professional appearance.
    (D) nonverbal communication.

7. The primary medical problem as defined by the patient is called

    (A) clinical history.
    (B) chief complaint.
    (C) subjective complaint.
    (D) objective complaint.

8. Which of the following would be considered examples of paralanguage?

    1. Diction
    2. Vocal pattern
    3. Fluency

    (A) 1 only
    (B) 2 only
    (C) 2 and 3 only
    (D) 1, 2, and 3

GO ON TO THE NEXT PAGE

KAPLAN

9. The most effective way to identify an inpatient waiting for a radiographic procedure is to

(A) call the patient by name.

(B) check the patient chart.

(C) establish a rapport with the patient in the waiting room.

(D) check the patient ID band after calling the patient's name.

Infection Control

1. According to the *Process of Infection*, the period between exposure to a disease-causing agent and the appearance of symptoms is known as

(A) incubation.

(B) latent.

(C) convalescence.

(D) prodromal.

2. Isolation techniques are a precise kind of

(A) germ control.

(B) sterilization.

(C) medical asepsis.

(D) surgical asepsis.

3. Hepatitis is an inflammatory disease of the

(A) kidneys.

(B) cystic duct.

(C) spleen.

(D) liver.

4. The medical term "enteric" means

(A) pertaining to the intestines.

(B) pertaining to disinfectant.

(C) standard precautions.

(D) therapeutic regimen.

5. A radiographer who performs frequent hand-washing to prevent the spread of infection would be applying

(A) surgical asepsis.

(B) medical asepsis.

(C) disinfection.

(D) sterilization.

6. Which of the following is a specific type of infection that a patient can acquire while being treated in the hospital, usually occurring within the first 72 hours of being admitted?

(A) Gangrene

(B) Sepsis

(C) Nosocomial

(D) TB

7. The exterior assembly of a chest-tube drainage device must always remain in which position?

(A) Lower than the patient's chest

(B) Higher than the patient's chest

(C) Level with the patient's chest

(D) Makes no difference where it is placed

8. In the operating room, the sterile corridor is between

(A) the anesthesiologist and the patient drape.

(B) the door and the patient drape.

(C) the patient drape and the surgeon.

(D) the patient drape and the instrument table.

9. When a sterile procedure tray is opened for a radiographic procedure, which flap of the sterile package will be opened LAST?

(A) The flap opened to the right

(B) The flap opened to the left

(C) The flap opened toward the radiographer

(D) The flap opened away from the radiographer

GO ON TO THE NEXT PAGE ▷

10. The complete removal of all microorganisms and their spores from the surface of an object is the definition of

    (A) surgical asepsis.
    (B) medical asepsis.
    (C) infection control.
    (D) isolation technique.

11. As the first step in the "Establishment of an Infectious Disease Process," an infectious organism comes in contact with the host. This is known as

    (A) damage.
    (B) outcome.
    (C) entry.
    (D) encounter.

12. In addition to standard precautions, the radiographer entering an isolation room of a patient with measles would adhere to which of the following precautions?

    (A) Reverse
    (B) Airborne
    (C) Droplet
    (D) Contact

13. If a patient is considered to be immunodepressed, he is

    (A) susceptible to infection.
    (B) contagious.
    (C) communicable.
    (D) infectious.

14. Which of the following is a disease-producing microorganism?

    (A) Bacteria
    (B) Fomite
    (C) Pathogen
    (D) Fungi

15. Vehicles that transport infectious microorganisms include

    (A) infectious secretions from the nose and mouth.
    (B) food, water, and blood contaminated with microorganisms.
    (C) insect and animal carriers of disease.
    (D) inanimate objects that harbor germs.

16. The standard length of time to perform a surgical scrub of the hands is

    (A) 2 minutes.
    (B) 4 minutes.
    (C) 6 minutes.
    (D) 10 minutes.

17. According to the *Guidelines for Environmental Infection Control in Health Care Facilities*, the EPA (Environmental Protection Agency) recommends that soiled areas of blood should be cleaned with which proportion of solution?

    (A) Chlorine bleach and water at a ratio of 1:1
    (B) Chlorine bleach and water at a ratio of 1:10
    (C) Chlorine bleach and water at a ratio of 1:50
    (D) Chlorine bleach and water at a ratio of 1:100

18. Strict aseptic technique is NOT a requirement of which of the following imaging procedures?

    (A) Myelogram
    (B) Arteriogram
    (C) Arthrogram
    (D) Barium enema

GO ON TO THE NEXT PAGE

KAPLAN

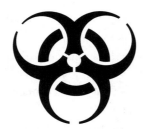

19. The figure above identifies which controlled area?

    (A) Radioactive
    (B) Magnetic
    (C) Nuclear
    (D) Biohazard

20. Which of the following is NOT one of the four factors included in the "Chain of Infection"?

    (A) A human host
    (B) The encounter
    (C) An infectious microorganism
    (D) The mode of transmission

21. Which of the following is the MOST common type of nosocomial infection?

    (A) Respiratory tract
    (B) Digestive tract
    (C) Alimentary tract
    (D) Urinary tract

22. An animal carrier that can transfer an infectious agent or disease from a host to another person is called which of the following?

    (A) Vector
    (B) Fomite
    (C) Fungi
    (D) Flora

23. According to correct procedure, a sterile radiographer would apply which of the following apparatus last?

    (A) Gloves
    (B) Gown
    (C) Face mask
    (D) Shoe covers

Physical Assistance and Transfer

1. A patient is having difficulty breathing while lying recumbent on the X-ray table. The patient should immediately be placed in which of the following positions?

    (A) Trendelenburg
    (B) Supine
    (C) Fowler's
    (D) Sims'

GO ON TO THE NEXT PAGE

Refer to the following figure for Question 2:

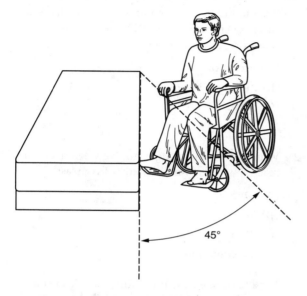

45°

2. The type of patient transfer demonstrated above is

(A) two-person lift transfer.

(B) parallel transfer.

(C) standby assist transfer.

(D) hydraulic lift transfer.

3. When helping a patient who has an Fx of the upper extremity to re-dress after the completion of a radiographic study,

(A) place the clothing on the patient's uninjured side first.

(B) place the clothing on the patient's injured side first.

(C) it makes no difference which arm is re-dressed first.

(D) allow the patient to choose which arm is re-dressed first.

4. Which of the following would NOT be considered good body mechanics for the radiographer when transferring a patient from a wheelchair to the X-ray table?

(A) Use a narrow base of support

(B) Bend at the knees when lifting

(C) Roll or push heavy objects

(D) Work at a comfortable height

5. The minimum number of radiographers that should be utilized to transfer a patient from the X-ray table to a stretcher without the use of a commercial moving device is

(A) one.

(B) two.

(C) three.

(D) four.

Medical Emergencies

1. Which of the following types of patient shock conditions would be due to an abnormally low circulating volume of blood or tissue fluids?

(A) Hypovolemic

(B) Cardiogenic

(C) Vasogenic

(D) Neurogenic

2. The medical term for the collapse of a lung is

(A) auscultation.

(B) purulent.

(C) atelectasis.

(D) intubation.

GO ON TO THE NEXT PAGE

3. The medical term that describes the light-headed feeling a patient may experience when moved from a recumbent to a standing position is

   (A) syncope.
   (B) CVA.
   (C) orthostatic hypotension.
   (D) vasovagal shock.

4. The medical term that describes a patient dependent upon daily insulin injections for diabetes mellitus is

   (A) gestational diabetic.
   (B) Type 1.
   (C) Type 2.
   (D) All of the above

5. On the Glasgow Coma Scale, which of the following scores would indicate that the patient has a very good prognosis for a full recovery from a severe brain injury?

   (A) 2
   (B) 6
   (C) 7
   (D) 14

6. The medical term for profuse sweating is

   (A) diaphoresis.
   (B) febrile.
   (C) epistaxis.
   (D) urticaria.

Contrast Media

1. Prior to radiographic contrast injection, lab tests checking creatinine and BUN levels are done to check the function of the

   (A) circulatory system.
   (B) endocrine system.
   (C) heart.
   (D) kidneys.

2. Which of the following is not considered a mild reaction to the administration of contrast?

   (A) Dizziness
   (B) Nausea
   (C) Pallor
   (D) Hypotension

3. For a barium enema procedure, the bag of contrast solution should be suspended above the patient by

   (A) 12".
   (B) 24".
   (C) 30".
   (D) 40".

4. A severe, life-threatening response to a drug or a contrast media is called

   (A) syncope.
   (B) lethargy.
   (C) epistaxis.
   (D) anaphylaxis.

5. The medical term "urticaria" means

   (A) nosebleed.
   (B) hives.
   (C) fainting.
   (D) difficulty swallowing.

GO ON TO THE NEXT PAGE ▷

6. The type of injection that will deliver a small amount of medication directly under the skin is which type of injection?

   (A) Venous

   (B) Intramuscular

   (C) Subcutaneous

   (D) Arterial

7. Of the procedures IVP, GB, GI, and BE, which should be scheduled LAST for the same patient?

   (A) IVP

   (B) GB

   (C) GI

   (D) BE

8. Which patient value is measured by pulse oximeter equipment?

   (A) Pulse only

   (B) Oxygen saturation only

   (C) Pulse and oxygen saturation

   (D) Pulse, oxygen saturation, and blood pressure

9. When performing venipuncture, what is the correct degree at which the needle should be inserted gently into the vein?

   (A) 10°

   (B) 15°

   (C) 20°

   (D) 45°

10. The intrathecal space surrounds which of the following structures?

    (A) Spinal cord

    (B) Brain

    (C) Knee joint

    (D) Heart

11. Which of the following needle sizes has the largest diameter?

    (A) 6 gauge

    (B) 14 gauge

    (C) 20 gauge

    (D) 28 gauge

12. During the injection of contrast media, the escape or discharge from a vein into the surrounding tissue is called

    (A) bolus.

    (B) IV push.

    (C) IV drip infusion.

    (D) infiltration.

13. Parenteral administration of a contrast media means that the contrast will be delivered by which of the following routes?

    (A) Enema

    (B) Orally

    (C) Injection

    (D) Nasogastric tube

14. Prior to radiographic contrast injection, normal creatinine blood lab values for an adult should be in which range?

    (A) 7 to 18 mg/dL

    (B) 170 to 240 mg/dL

    (C) 0.6 to 1.3 mg/dL

    (D) 1.6 to 7.0 mg/dL

15. What is the medical abbreviation for two times per day?

    (A) BID

    (B) TID

    (C) QID

    (D) PRN

GO ON TO THE NEXT PAGE

KAPLAN

Refer to the following figure for Questions 16 and 17:

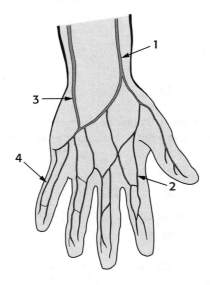

16. In the figure above, the vein identified by the Number 3 is the

(A) cephalic.
(B) accessory cephalic.
(C) median cubital.
(D) basilic.

17. The vein identified by the Number 1 is the

(A) cephalic.
(B) accessory cephalic.
(C) median cubital.
(D) basilic.

Answers and Explanations

Ethical and Legal Aspects

1. The correct answer is (A).

False imprisonment is defined as the unjustifiable detention of a person against his or her will. The radiographer must follow hospital policy, which includes using restraints only when ordered by a physician.

2. The correct answer is (D).

Radiology patient data sheets are legal documents and must include the patient name, patient history, and the name of the radiographer performing the examination.

3. The correct answer is (A).

The definition of autonomy is that patients are treated as individuals and are informed about procedures so they will have the appropriate information to make decisions in their own care. Both the living will and durable power of attorney are advance directives.

4. The correct answer is (C).

A consent form must be signed by the patient, patient guardian, or designee to be valid. So if the consent to treat a minor was signed by the treating physician and not the parent or guardian, this would qualify it as the incorrect choice.

5. The correct answer is (D).

Slander is defined as the verbal or oral spreading of malicious information that damages the reputation of another individual. Libel (C) refers to a written assault or defamation of an individual. Medical negligence (B) is a failure to follow the appropriate standard of care that results in harm to a patient. Malpractice (A) may be found when harm is caused to a patient that results when health care workers do not follow appropriate standards of care and medical negligence is found.

6. The correct answer is (C).

The radiographer may be charged with battery, defined as the unlawful touching of a person without consent. It is important that the radiographer communicate with the patient, especially before touching and positioning the patient, to avoid any miscommunication during a radiographic procedure.

7. The correct answer is (B).

Veracity is the obligation to tell the truth and not to deceive others. Autonomy (A), within patient care, provides that patients are informed about procedures so that they will have the appropriate information to make decisions about their own care. Statutory disclosure (C) requires that medical professionals and institutions, depending on state law, report certain medical conditions and incidents.

8. The correct answer is (D).

A Living Will, a DNR (Do Not Resuscitate) order, and a DNI (Do Not Intubate) order are all examples of advance health care directives. Advance health care directives are documents completed by patients, while they have autonomy (decision-making ability), to choose someone to make decisions for them should they become unable to make their own medical decisions. To be legal, all advance health care directives must be in writing, signed, and witnessed.

9. The correct answer is (A).

Nonmaleficence means "do no harm." It refers to a radiographer's duty to refrain from doing harm to a patient, and to the radiographer's obligation to maintain a professional standard of care at all times.

10. The correct answer is (D).

The legal theory or doctrine of "Respondeat Superior" means the master speaks for the servant. It applies that in some circumstances, the employer may be held responsible for the actions of the employee. Res ipsa loquitur (A) means "the thing speaks for itself."

11. The correct answer is (D).

A charge of medical malpractice may be brought against a radiographer who fails to provide the applicable standard of care to the patient if the result is injury or harm to the patient. Battery (A) is the unlawful touching of a person without consent. A tort (C) is a subdivision of civil law used to recover damages occurring from negligent conduct.

12. The correct answer is (B).

The key focus of the Health Insurance Portability and Accountability Act of 1996 (HIPAA) is the confidentiality, privacy, and security of patient health information and records.

13. The correct answer is (B).

A DNR order, also known as a Do Not Resuscitate order or "no code," alerts health care workers that if death is imminent the patient has chosen that no effort at emergency resuscitation is to be attempted. DNI (C) is a Do Not Intubate order. Both the DNR and DNI order are advance directives that must be expressed by the patient in the event the patient loses the ability to communicate on his or her own behalf. DRG (A) stands for Diagnosis-Related Group.

14. The correct answer is (D).

A tort is a subdivision of the law that allows for the recovery of damages for acts of negligence or personal injury. Torts are the most common type of lawsuit filed against radiographers for charges of assault, battery, false imprisonment, medical malpractice, and breach of patient confidentiality.

15. The correct answer is (D).

All of the following are included in the Patient's Bill of Rights: the patient has the right to considerate and respectful care; the patient has the right to every consideration of privacy; and the patient has the right to have an advance directive (a living will, health care proxy, or durable power of attorney for health care).

Interpersonal Communication

1. The correct answer is (C).

Dr. Kübler-Ross's theory of the grieving process states that the five steps that patients will go through as an emotional response to loss, in order, are: denial, anger, bargaining, depression, and acceptance.

2. The correct answer is (C).

A subjective finding is something that the patient tells you is happening. Objective findings are actual data or test results that can be recorded. An objective finding would be a blood test or palpated mass that can be felt or measured.

3. The correct answer is (A).

Blind patients communicate mostly through verbal communication. Instructions for blind patients should be clear and supportive. The radiographer should clearly let the patient know what is expected of him and guide him with a gentle touch when appropriate.

4. The correct answer is (A).

Empathy is the ability to enter into a patient's feelings. Having empathy allows a radiographer to be more compassionate. It is different from having sympathy or pity for the patient. Rapport is building harmony and a relationship with a patient.

5. The correct answer is (C).

Communication is the key to successful patient interactions. It will reduce voluntary patient motion, and therefore the number of repeats necessary. Taking a few minutes for explanation and demonstration will ensure an optimal study.

6. The correct answer is (D).

Nonverbal communication includes communicating with the patient in forms other than words, and is important for effective patient interaction. Nonverbal communication includes eye contact, body language, palpation, and professional appearance.

7. The correct answer is (B).

The primary medical problem as defined by the patient during a physical exam is termed the chief complaint. The chief complaint will focus the clinical history toward the single most important issue.

8. The correct answer is (D).

All of the items listed would be considered examples of paralanguage (the rhythm of speech).

9. The correct answer is (D).

The radiographer should call the patient by name and check the ID band to ensure it is the correct patient. Checking the patient ID band is a necessary practice, and must be done for all inpatients.

Infection Control

1. The correct answer is (B).

The latent period during the process of infection defines the time between the exposure to a disease and the appearance of symptoms. Incubation (A) is the period when pathogens enter and no symptoms exist. Convalescence (C) is the recovery stage, when symptoms diminish. Prodromal (D) is the highly infectious period.

2. The correct answer is (C).

All patient isolation techniques follow the rules of medical asepsis. It is important that the radiographer follow hospital protocol when entering patient isolation rooms. Hand-washing, gloves, masks, and room isolation are all forms of medical asepsis to protect both the patient and technologist.

3. The correct answer is (D).

Hepatitis is an inflammation of the liver.

4. The correct answer is (A).

The medical term "enteric" means pertaining to the intestines.

5. The correct answer is (B).

Hand-washing is a type of medical asepsis used to prevent the spread of infection. The radiographer should wash his or her hands before and after touching each patient so as not to spread infection.

6. The correct answer is (C).

A nosocomial infection is a specific type of infection that is acquired while a patient is receiving care while in the hospital. Nosocomial infections can best be prevented when good medial asepsis is practiced by all health care workers.

7. The correct answer is (A).

The exterior assembly of a chest-tube drainage device must always remain lower than the patient's chest; this way, fluid is prevented from flowing backward and causing an infection.

8. The correct answer is (D).

The sterile corridor is the area between the patient drape and the instrument table in the operating room. In the operating room, the radiographer must be certain to pay strict attention to sterile procedures at all times.

9. The correct answer is (C).

The correct order for opening a sterile pack is as follows:
In Step 1, the first flap is opened away from the radiographer. In Steps 2 and 3, the flaps are opened to the right and the left. In Step 4, the last flap is opened toward the radiographer.

10. The correct answer is (A).

Surgical asepsis is the complete removal of the microorganisms and their spores from the surface of an object. Medical asepsis (B) is the practice that will reduce the number of microorganisms to as few as possible.

11. The correct answer is (D).

The six steps of the establishment of infectious disease, in order, are: encounter, entry, spread, multiplication, damage, and outcome.

12. The correct answer is (B).

In addition to applying standard precautions, the radiographer entering the isolation room of a patient with measles would also apply airborne precaution procedures.

13. The correct answer is (A).

Patients who are immunodepressed may not be able to defend themselves from opportunistic infections. This condition may be due to poor health or the result of medical treatment. The patient is in a weakened state and unable to fight off disease and opportunistic infections.

14. The correct answer is (C).

A pathogen is defined as any disease-producing microorganism. Bacteria (A) are microscopic single-celled organisms. Fomite (B) are inanimate objects that cannot do harm but can harbor germs. Fungi (D) are macroscopic yeasts and molds.

15. The correct answer is (B).

A vehicle route of transport of infectious microorganisms includes food, water, drugs, and blood contaminated with microorganisms. Infectious secretions from the nose and mouth (A) is droplet contact. Vectors are insect and animal carriers of disease (C). Inanimate objects that can harbor germs are fomites (D).

16. The correct answer is (D).

17. The correct answer is (B).

According to the guidelines, the EPA recommends that areas of patient surface contact (such as an X-ray table soiled with blood) should be cleaned with a solution of 1 part chlorine bleach to 10 parts water.

18. The correct answer is (D).

A barium enema procedure is done under non-aseptic technique conditions. The other choices are all radiographic studies that require an injection and would require aseptic technique.

19. The correct answer is (D).

The figure identifies an area of biohazard.

20. The correct answer is (B).

The encounter is not part of the chain of infection. The four factors linked in the spread of disease are human host, reservoir, infectious microorganism, and mode of transmission.

21. The correct answer is (D).

A urinary tract infection is the most common type of nosocomial acquired infection. A nosocomial infection is a type of infection that is acquired while a patient is receiving care in the hospital. Nosocomial infections can best be prevented with proper medical asepsis practiced at all times by health care workers.

22. The correct answer is (A).

A vector is an animal that can transfer an infectious agent or disease from a host to another person. Fomites (B) are inanimate objects such as radiographic tables or cassettes that can harbor germs. Fungi (C) is a general term for a group of yeasts and molds. Flora (D) are part of the microbial community routinely found on parts of the healthy human body.

23. The correct answer is (A).

The radiographer must follow strict sterile procedure at all times when working in the OR area. That means he would put on the gloves last after the shoe covers, mask, and gown. Hospital protocols should be followed at all times to maintain a sterile environment in the OR.

Physical Assistance and Transfer

1. The correct answer is (C).

A patient who has difficulty breathing when lying recumbent should be moved to a stretcher right away and placed in the Fowler's position. This will raise his head to an angle of 45 to 90° and allow him to breathe more easily. Trendelenburg (A) is where the patient's head is lower than his feet. Sims' (D) is an oblique recumbent patient position.

2. The correct answer is (C).

A standby assist transfer is demonstrated in the image.

3. The correct answer is (B).

After completing a radiographic study, when assisting someone to re-dress who has an Fx (fracture) of the upper extremity, it is best to place the clothing on the patient's injured side first. It will be easier to move the clothing around the injured extremity if it is placed on the injured arm first.

4. The correct choice is (A).

A narrow base of support is the improper use of body mechanics. The radiographer should use a broad base of support when transferring a patient from a wheelchair to the X-ray table; this prevents bending and twisting of the back (a common injury among health care workers). Bending at the knees, rolling or pushing heavy objects, working at a comfortable height, and keeping the back straight when lifting are all rules to be followed for maintaining proper body mechanics.

5. The correct choice is (C).

Correct procedure dictates that if no commercial moving device is to be used, at least three people must assist when transferring a patient from the X-ray table to a stretcher.

Medical Emergencies

1. The correct answer is (A).

Hypovolemic shock is a type of patient shock that results from an abnormally low circulating volume of blood or tissue fluids. The decrease in blood and fluids may be due to trauma or post-surgical complication. Cardiogenic shock (B) is due to cardiac disorders and a failure of the heart to work properly. Vasogenic shock (C) is due to sepsis, severe allergic reactions, and anesthesia. Neurogenic shock (D) is due to brain injury and spinal anesthesia.

2. The correct answer is (C).

Atelectasis is defined as the collapse of a lung. Auscultation (A) is the sound produced by the structures of the lungs during breathing. Purulent (B) is the medical term for pus. Intubation (D) is the passage of a tube into the trachea to ensure breathing.

3. The correct answer is (C).

Orthostatic hypotension is the rapid drop in blood pressure caused when a patient stands too quickly or sits up too suddenly after lying in bed for a long period of time. Syncope (A) means fainting. A CVA (B) is a cerebral vascular accident (stroke), which is the rupture of a cerebral artery in the brain. Vasovagal shock (D) is a type of shock or failure of the circulatory system to support body functions.

4. The correct answer is (B).

Type 1 diabetic patients are dependent upon daily insulin injections. Type 2 diabetes (C) is usually controlled through diet and exercise but must be checked regularly. Gestational diabetes (A) occurs in the later months of pregnancy and is usually treated with diet.

5. The correct answer is (C).

The high score of 14 on the Glasgow Coma Scale indicates that the patient has an excellent chance of a full recovery. The Glasgow Scale is used to observe the patient in three areas: eyes opening, motor response, and verbal response, with a maximum rating of 15 points. Since this patient scored 14 out of a possible 15 points, the prognosis is excellent.

6. The correct answer is (A).

Diaphoresis is the medical term for profuse sweating, which is a way for the body to dissipate heat. Epistaxis (C) means nosebleed, and urticaria (D) is hives.

Contrast Media

1. The correct answer is (D).

Lab tests are done prior to a radiographic procedure that will require an injection of contrast media. BUN and creatinine tests check the function of the kidneys, because that is where the contrast media will be excreted.

2. The correct answer is (D).

Hypotension, which is the decrease in blood pressure of the patient, would not be considered a mild reaction to the effects of the administration of contrast media. A hypotensive reaction is considered a moderate reaction. All of the remaining answer choices are mild reactions.

3. The correct answer is (C).

For a barium enema, the bag containing the barium solution should be suspended at least 30″ above the patient so that the solution in the bag will be able to flow freely.

4. The correct answer is (D).

Anaphylaxis is a type of shock that is severe, progresses quickly, and may be life-threatening. It may be an allergic reaction or a response to a drug or a contrast media administered as part of an X-ray exam. Syncope (A) means fainting. Epistaxis (C) means nosebleed.

5. The correct answer is (B).

The medical term for urticaria is hives.

6. The correct answer is (C).

A subcutaneous injection is one that will deliver the medication directly below the surface of the skin into the subcutaneous tissue.

7. The correct answer is (C).

The upper GI exam would be scheduled last. When a patient is to be scheduled for multiple contrast procedures that involve intravascular contrast agents, such as the IVP, would be scheduled first. Intravascular contrast is less dense than barium. Lower GI studies are done before upper GI studies. Upper GI exams are scheduled last.

8. The correct answer is (C).

Pulse oximeter equipment is used to measure the patient's pulse rate and blood oxygen values. Blood pressure is not measured with a pulse oximeter.

9. The correct answer is (B).

When performing venipuncture, the needle should be inserted gently into the vein at an angle of 15°.

10. The correct answer is (A).

The intrathecal space is the area around the spinal cord. This area may be used to administer high, local concentrations of drugs for pain relief, and for contrast administration during certain radiology procedures.

11. The correct answer is (A).

The needle with the smallest number gauge will have the largest diameter.

12. The correct answer is (D).

The escape or discharge from a vein into the surrounding tissue during the actual injection is called an infiltration. An infiltration is also called an extravasation and must be treated immediately.

13. The correct answer is (C).

Parenteral administration of a contrast medium or drug means that the solution will be given by injection or via a route other than the gastrointestinal tract.

14. The correct answer is (C).

The correct value range is 0.6 to 1.3 mg/dL. For an adult patient, a normal creatinine blood lab value taken prior to radiographic contrast studies should fall in this range.

15. The correct answer is (A).

The medical abbreviation that means two times per day is BID. The other terms are: TID (B), three times per day; QID (C), four times per day; and PRN (D), as needed.

16. The correct answer is (D).

On the hand diagram, the vein identified by Number 3 is the basilic vein.

17. The correct answer is (A).

The vein identified by Number 1 is the cephalic vein.

PART THREE

Full-Length Practice Test

HOW TO TAKE THE PRACTICE TESTS

Before taking the tests, find a quiet place where you can work for three hours. Make sure you have a comfortable desk and several pencils. Keep in mind that the real ARRT exam is given on computer, so its format for answering questions will vary a bit from those seen here.

Once you have started the practice test, don't stop until you have gone through the entire exam. It is to your advantage to answer every question, because no points are deducted for wrong answers. In fact, the computer will not proceed unless you indicate some response to every question.

Good luck on the exam!

1 Ⓐ Ⓑ Ⓒ Ⓓ	51 Ⓐ Ⓑ Ⓒ Ⓓ	101 Ⓐ Ⓑ Ⓒ Ⓓ	151 Ⓐ Ⓑ Ⓒ Ⓓ
2 Ⓐ Ⓑ Ⓒ Ⓓ	52 Ⓐ Ⓑ Ⓒ Ⓓ	102 Ⓐ Ⓑ Ⓒ Ⓓ	152 Ⓐ Ⓑ Ⓒ Ⓓ
3 Ⓐ Ⓑ Ⓒ Ⓓ	53 Ⓐ Ⓑ Ⓒ Ⓓ	103 Ⓐ Ⓑ Ⓒ Ⓓ	153 Ⓐ Ⓑ Ⓒ Ⓓ
4 Ⓐ Ⓑ Ⓒ Ⓓ	54 Ⓐ Ⓑ Ⓒ Ⓓ	104 Ⓐ Ⓑ Ⓒ Ⓓ	154 Ⓐ Ⓑ Ⓒ Ⓓ
5 Ⓐ Ⓑ Ⓒ Ⓓ	55 Ⓐ Ⓑ Ⓒ Ⓓ	105 Ⓐ Ⓑ Ⓒ Ⓓ	155 Ⓐ Ⓑ Ⓒ Ⓓ
6 Ⓐ Ⓑ Ⓒ Ⓓ	56 Ⓐ Ⓑ Ⓒ Ⓓ	106 Ⓐ Ⓑ Ⓒ Ⓓ	156 Ⓐ Ⓑ Ⓒ Ⓓ
7 Ⓐ Ⓑ Ⓒ Ⓓ	57 Ⓐ Ⓑ Ⓒ Ⓓ	107 Ⓐ Ⓑ Ⓒ Ⓓ	157 Ⓐ Ⓑ Ⓒ Ⓓ
8 Ⓐ Ⓑ Ⓒ Ⓓ	58 Ⓐ Ⓑ Ⓒ Ⓓ	108 Ⓐ Ⓑ Ⓒ Ⓓ	158 Ⓐ Ⓑ Ⓒ Ⓓ
9 Ⓐ Ⓑ Ⓒ Ⓓ	59 Ⓐ Ⓑ Ⓒ Ⓓ	109 Ⓐ Ⓑ Ⓒ Ⓓ	159 Ⓐ Ⓑ Ⓒ Ⓓ
10 Ⓐ Ⓑ Ⓒ Ⓓ	60 Ⓐ Ⓑ Ⓒ Ⓓ	110 Ⓐ Ⓑ Ⓒ Ⓓ	160 Ⓐ Ⓑ Ⓒ Ⓓ
11 Ⓐ Ⓑ Ⓒ Ⓓ	61 Ⓐ Ⓑ Ⓒ Ⓓ	111 Ⓐ Ⓑ Ⓒ Ⓓ	161 Ⓐ Ⓑ Ⓒ Ⓓ
12 Ⓐ Ⓑ Ⓒ Ⓓ	62 Ⓐ Ⓑ Ⓒ Ⓓ	112 Ⓐ Ⓑ Ⓒ Ⓓ	162 Ⓐ Ⓑ Ⓒ Ⓓ
13 Ⓐ Ⓑ Ⓒ Ⓓ	63 Ⓐ Ⓑ Ⓒ Ⓓ	113 Ⓐ Ⓑ Ⓒ Ⓓ	163 Ⓐ Ⓑ Ⓒ Ⓓ
14 Ⓐ Ⓑ Ⓒ Ⓓ	64 Ⓐ Ⓑ Ⓒ Ⓓ	114 Ⓐ Ⓑ Ⓒ Ⓓ	164 Ⓐ Ⓑ Ⓒ Ⓓ
15 Ⓐ Ⓑ Ⓒ Ⓓ	65 Ⓐ Ⓑ Ⓒ Ⓓ	115 Ⓐ Ⓑ Ⓒ Ⓓ	165 Ⓐ Ⓑ Ⓒ Ⓓ
16 Ⓐ Ⓑ Ⓒ Ⓓ	66 Ⓐ Ⓑ Ⓒ Ⓓ	116 Ⓐ Ⓑ Ⓒ Ⓓ	166 Ⓐ Ⓑ Ⓒ Ⓓ
17 Ⓐ Ⓑ Ⓒ Ⓓ	67 Ⓐ Ⓑ Ⓒ Ⓓ	117 Ⓐ Ⓑ Ⓒ Ⓓ	167 Ⓐ Ⓑ Ⓒ Ⓓ
18 Ⓐ Ⓑ Ⓒ Ⓓ	68 Ⓐ Ⓑ Ⓒ Ⓓ	118 Ⓐ Ⓑ Ⓒ Ⓓ	168 Ⓐ Ⓑ Ⓒ Ⓓ
19 Ⓐ Ⓑ Ⓒ Ⓓ	69 Ⓐ Ⓑ Ⓒ Ⓓ	119 Ⓐ Ⓑ Ⓒ Ⓓ	169 Ⓐ Ⓑ Ⓒ Ⓓ
20 Ⓐ Ⓑ Ⓒ Ⓓ	70 Ⓐ Ⓑ Ⓒ Ⓓ	120 Ⓐ Ⓑ Ⓒ Ⓓ	170 Ⓐ Ⓑ Ⓒ Ⓓ
21 Ⓐ Ⓑ Ⓒ Ⓓ	71 Ⓐ Ⓑ Ⓒ Ⓓ	121 Ⓐ Ⓑ Ⓒ Ⓓ	171 Ⓐ Ⓑ Ⓒ Ⓓ
22 Ⓐ Ⓑ Ⓒ Ⓓ	72 Ⓐ Ⓑ Ⓒ Ⓓ	122 Ⓐ Ⓑ Ⓒ Ⓓ	172 Ⓐ Ⓑ Ⓒ Ⓓ
23 Ⓐ Ⓑ Ⓒ Ⓓ	73 Ⓐ Ⓑ Ⓒ Ⓓ	123 Ⓐ Ⓑ Ⓒ Ⓓ	173 Ⓐ Ⓑ Ⓒ Ⓓ
24 Ⓐ Ⓑ Ⓒ Ⓓ	74 Ⓐ Ⓑ Ⓒ Ⓓ	124 Ⓐ Ⓑ Ⓒ Ⓓ	174 Ⓐ Ⓑ Ⓒ Ⓓ
25 Ⓐ Ⓑ Ⓒ Ⓓ	75 Ⓐ Ⓑ Ⓒ Ⓓ	125 Ⓐ Ⓑ Ⓒ Ⓓ	175 Ⓐ Ⓑ Ⓒ Ⓓ
26 Ⓐ Ⓑ Ⓒ Ⓓ	76 Ⓐ Ⓑ Ⓒ Ⓓ	126 Ⓐ Ⓑ Ⓒ Ⓓ	176 Ⓐ Ⓑ Ⓒ Ⓓ
27 Ⓐ Ⓑ Ⓒ Ⓓ	77 Ⓐ Ⓑ Ⓒ Ⓓ	127 Ⓐ Ⓑ Ⓒ Ⓓ	177 Ⓐ Ⓑ Ⓒ Ⓓ
28 Ⓐ Ⓑ Ⓒ Ⓓ	78 Ⓐ Ⓑ Ⓒ Ⓓ	128 Ⓐ Ⓑ Ⓒ Ⓓ	178 Ⓐ Ⓑ Ⓒ Ⓓ
29 Ⓐ Ⓑ Ⓒ Ⓓ	79 Ⓐ Ⓑ Ⓒ Ⓓ	129 Ⓐ Ⓑ Ⓒ Ⓓ	179 Ⓐ Ⓑ Ⓒ Ⓓ
30 Ⓐ Ⓑ Ⓒ Ⓓ	80 Ⓐ Ⓑ Ⓒ Ⓓ	130 Ⓐ Ⓑ Ⓒ Ⓓ	180 Ⓐ Ⓑ Ⓒ Ⓓ
31 Ⓐ Ⓑ Ⓒ Ⓓ	81 Ⓐ Ⓑ Ⓒ Ⓓ	131 Ⓐ Ⓑ Ⓒ Ⓓ	181 Ⓐ Ⓑ Ⓒ Ⓓ
32 Ⓐ Ⓑ Ⓒ Ⓓ	82 Ⓐ Ⓑ Ⓒ Ⓓ	132 Ⓐ Ⓑ Ⓒ Ⓓ	182 Ⓐ Ⓑ Ⓒ Ⓓ
33 Ⓐ Ⓑ Ⓒ Ⓓ	83 Ⓐ Ⓑ Ⓒ Ⓓ	133 Ⓐ Ⓑ Ⓒ Ⓓ	183 Ⓐ Ⓑ Ⓒ Ⓓ
34 Ⓐ Ⓑ Ⓒ Ⓓ	84 Ⓐ Ⓑ Ⓒ Ⓓ	134 Ⓐ Ⓑ Ⓒ Ⓓ	184 Ⓐ Ⓑ Ⓒ Ⓓ
35 Ⓐ Ⓑ Ⓒ Ⓓ	85 Ⓐ Ⓑ Ⓒ Ⓓ	135 Ⓐ Ⓑ Ⓒ Ⓓ	185 Ⓐ Ⓑ Ⓒ Ⓓ
36 Ⓐ Ⓑ Ⓒ Ⓓ	86 Ⓐ Ⓑ Ⓒ Ⓓ	136 Ⓐ Ⓑ Ⓒ Ⓓ	186 Ⓐ Ⓑ Ⓒ Ⓓ
37 Ⓐ Ⓑ Ⓒ Ⓓ	87 Ⓐ Ⓑ Ⓒ Ⓓ	137 Ⓐ Ⓑ Ⓒ Ⓓ	187 Ⓐ Ⓑ Ⓒ Ⓓ
38 Ⓐ Ⓑ Ⓒ Ⓓ	88 Ⓐ Ⓑ Ⓒ Ⓓ	138 Ⓐ Ⓑ Ⓒ Ⓓ	188 Ⓐ Ⓑ Ⓒ Ⓓ
39 Ⓐ Ⓑ Ⓒ Ⓓ	89 Ⓐ Ⓑ Ⓒ Ⓓ	139 Ⓐ Ⓑ Ⓒ Ⓓ	189 Ⓐ Ⓑ Ⓒ Ⓓ
40 Ⓐ Ⓑ Ⓒ Ⓓ	90 Ⓐ Ⓑ Ⓒ Ⓓ	140 Ⓐ Ⓑ Ⓒ Ⓓ	190 Ⓐ Ⓑ Ⓒ Ⓓ
41 Ⓐ Ⓑ Ⓒ Ⓓ	91 Ⓐ Ⓑ Ⓒ Ⓓ	141 Ⓐ Ⓑ Ⓒ Ⓓ	191 Ⓐ Ⓑ Ⓒ Ⓓ
42 Ⓐ Ⓑ Ⓒ Ⓓ	92 Ⓐ Ⓑ Ⓒ Ⓓ	142 Ⓐ Ⓑ Ⓒ Ⓓ	192 Ⓐ Ⓑ Ⓒ Ⓓ
43 Ⓐ Ⓑ Ⓒ Ⓓ	93 Ⓐ Ⓑ Ⓒ Ⓓ	143 Ⓐ Ⓑ Ⓒ Ⓓ	193 Ⓐ Ⓑ Ⓒ Ⓓ
44 Ⓐ Ⓑ Ⓒ Ⓓ	94 Ⓐ Ⓑ Ⓒ Ⓓ	144 Ⓐ Ⓑ Ⓒ Ⓓ	194 Ⓐ Ⓑ Ⓒ Ⓓ
45 Ⓐ Ⓑ Ⓒ Ⓓ	95 Ⓐ Ⓑ Ⓒ Ⓓ	145 Ⓐ Ⓑ Ⓒ Ⓓ	195 Ⓐ Ⓑ Ⓒ Ⓓ
46 Ⓐ Ⓑ Ⓒ Ⓓ	96 Ⓐ Ⓑ Ⓒ Ⓓ	146 Ⓐ Ⓑ Ⓒ Ⓓ	196 Ⓐ Ⓑ Ⓒ Ⓓ
47 Ⓐ Ⓑ Ⓒ Ⓓ	97 Ⓐ Ⓑ Ⓒ Ⓓ	147 Ⓐ Ⓑ Ⓒ Ⓓ	197 Ⓐ Ⓑ Ⓒ Ⓓ
48 Ⓐ Ⓑ Ⓒ Ⓓ	98 Ⓐ Ⓑ Ⓒ Ⓓ	148 Ⓐ Ⓑ Ⓒ Ⓓ	198 Ⓐ Ⓑ Ⓒ Ⓓ
49 Ⓐ Ⓑ Ⓒ Ⓓ	99 Ⓐ Ⓑ Ⓒ Ⓓ	149 Ⓐ Ⓑ Ⓒ Ⓓ	199 Ⓐ Ⓑ Ⓒ Ⓓ
50 Ⓐ Ⓑ Ⓒ Ⓓ	100 Ⓐ Ⓑ Ⓒ Ⓓ	150 Ⓐ Ⓑ Ⓒ Ⓓ	200 Ⓐ Ⓑ Ⓒ Ⓓ

Practice Test

Directions: For each of the following questions, choose the best answer given. Mark your answers in the answer grid (on the real exam, you will be clicking an oval on the computer screen).

1. The only direct articulation between the upper limbs and the trunk of the body is the

   (A) sternoclavicular joints.
   (B) acrominoclavicular joints.
   (C) manubriosternal joints.
   (D) costovertebral joints.

2. Which of the following positions of the chest demonstrate air-fluid levels to diagnose the presence of pleural effusion?

   1. Erect
   2. Supine
   3. Decubitus

   (A) 1 only
   (B) 1 and 3 only
   (C) 2 and 3 only
   (D) 1, 2, and 3

3. Which of the following is the correct sequencing of thoracic structures from anterior to posterior?

   1. Heart
   2. Descending aorta
   3. Proximal esophagus
   4. Trachea

   (A) 1, 2, 3, 4
   (B) 1, 4, 3, 2
   (C) 2, 3, 1, 4
   (D) 3, 1, 2, 4

KAPLAN

Refer to the following image for Question 4:

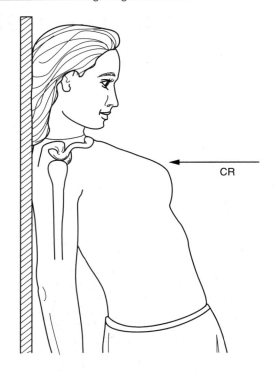

CR

4. The position being demonstrated above will best visualize which portion of the lungs on the image?

(A) The costophrenic angles

(B) The cardiophrenic angles

(C) The area above the clavicles

(D) The area beneath the clavicles

5. Which of the following is TRUE when positioning the patient for the lateral chest radiograph?

(A) Midcoronal plane is perpendicular to image receptor, central ray to level of T7

(B) Midcoronal plane is parallel to image receptor, central ray to level of T7

(C) Midsagittal plane is perpendicular to image receptor, central ray to level of T3

(D) Midsagittal plane is parallel to image receptor, central ray to level of T3

6. For the body rotation method of positioning for sternoclavicular joints, which of the following positions will BEST visualize the left sternoclavicular joint on the radiographic image?

(A) 15° RAO

(B) 15° LAO

(C) 30° RAO

(D) 30° LAO

7. The condition in which the nerves controlling rhythmic contractions of the large intestine are missing is called

(A) atresia.

(B) celiac disease.

(C) Hirschsprung disease.

(D) volvulus.

8. During a small bowel series, radiographs taken with the patient in which of the following positions will help to compress the abdominal contents, thereby increasing radiographic quality?

(A) Supine

(B) Prone

(C) Trendelenburg

(D) Lateral decubitus

9. When performing an upper gastrointestinal series, for the AP projection of the stomach and duodenum, the central ray is directed to which level on the average patient?

(A) T7

(B) T10

(C) L1

(D) L5

GO ON TO THE NEXT PAGE

10. Which of the following studies of the alimentary canal require that images be taken at timed intervals?

    1. Upper GI series
    2. Small bowel series
    3. Enteroclysis procedure

(A) 1 only

(B) 2 only

(C) 1 and 3 only

(D) 2 and 3 only

Refer to the following image for Questions 11 to 13:

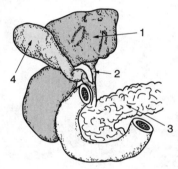

11. Which arrow identifies the organ that manufactures bile?

(A) 1

(B) 2

(C) 3

(D) 4

12. The structure being identified by Arrow 2 is the

(A) common bile duct.

(B) common hepatic duct.

(C) cystic duct.

(D) pancreatic duct.

13. Which numbered organ functions as both an endocrine and an exocrine gland?

(A) 1

(B) 2

(C) 3

(D) 4

14. Which decubitus position best demonstrates free air within the abdomen?

(A) Right lateral

(B) Left lateral

(C) Ventral

(D) Dorsal

15. Which of the following is the average body build?

(A) Asthenic

(B) Hypersthenic

(C) Hyposthenic

(D) Sthenic

Refer to the following radiograph for Questions 16 and 17:

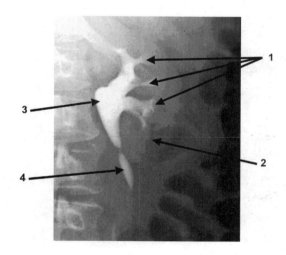

16. Which arrow identifies the renal calyces?

(A) 1

(B) 2

(C) 3

(D) 4

GO ON TO THE NEXT PAGE

17. Which arrow identifies the ureter?

    (A) 1

    (B) 2

    (C) 3

    (D) 4

18. Which of the following blood chemistry levels should be reviewed prior to contrast injection for intravenous urography?

    1. BUN
    2. Creatinine
    3. Hemoglobin

    (A) 1 only

    (B) 1 and 2 only

    (C) 2 and 3 only

    (D) 1, 2, and 3

19. The body position that BEST demonstrates positional change of the kidneys is

    (A) AP, supine.

    (B) AP erect, post-void.

    (C) AP, Trendelenburg.

    (D) obliques.

20. The central ray is directed to which level for an AP pelvis?

    (A) Iliac crests

    (B) ASIS (anterior superior iliac spines)

    (C) Midway between ASISs and pubic symphysis

    (D) Pubic symphysis

21. A rheumatic condition of the spine causing rigidity and fusing of the joints is

    (A) anklyosing spondylitis.

    (B) herniated nucleus pulposus.

    (C) spina bifida.

    (D) scoliosis.

22. If the cervicothoracic region is not well visualized on a lateral thoracic spine image, which of the following will better demonstrate that area?

    (A) Flexion, extension

    (B) Lateral, swimmers

    (C) Cross-table lateral, cervical spine

    (D) Lateral thoracic, breathing technique

Refer to the following radiograph for Questions 23 and 24:

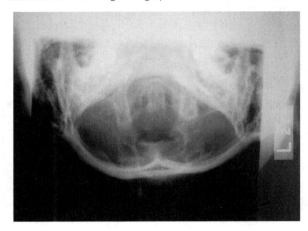

23. With the patient in the prone position, what is the angle of the OML in relation to the plane of the image receptor for positioning of the radiograph above?

    (A) 15°

    (B) 30°

    (C) 37°

    (D) 55°

24. The extension of the neck required for the positioning of the radiograph above is contraindicated for which of the following cases?

    1. Degenerative cervical disease
    2. Unhealed fracture
    3. Cervical collar

    (A) 1 only

    (B) 1 and 3 only

    (C) 2 and 3 only

    (D) 1, 2, and 3

GO ON TO THE NEXT PAGE

Refer to the following image for Questions 25 and 26:

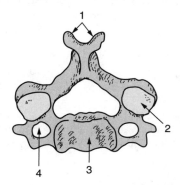

Refer to the following radiograph for Questions 28 and 29:

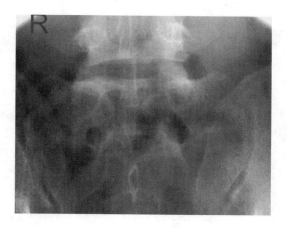

25. The figure above represents which type of vertebra?

(A) Cervical

(B) Thoracic

(C) Lumbar

(D) Sacral

26. The zygapophyseal joints are formed at the portion identified by which arrow?

(A) 1

(B) 2

(C) 3

(D) 4

27. Which of the following should be the first image acquired for the cervical spine procedure of a trauma patient?

(A) AP axial

(B) AP (Fuchs)

(C) Obliques

(D) Cross-table lateral

28. For a male patient that is supine, what is the correct central ray angle to produce the radiograph above?

(A) 15° cephalad

(B) 15° caudad

(C) 30° cephalad

(D) 30° caudad

29. The positioning utilized to produce this radiograph is the same as which of the following AP projections?

(A) Sacrum

(B) Sacroiliac joints

(C) Coccyx

(D) Acetabulum

GO ON TO THE NEXT PAGE

KAPLAN

Refer to the following image for Questions 30 and 31:

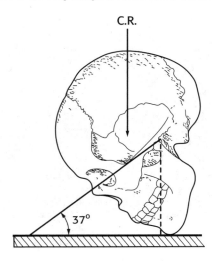

C.R.

37°

30. When the positioning demonstrated in the figure above is utilized, where will the petrous ridges appear on the image?

(A) Filling the orbits

(B) Upper two-thirds of orbits

(C) Lower one-third of orbits

(D) Below the maxillary sinuses

31. The positioning demonstrated, prone or erect, can be utilized for visualization of which of the following structures?

   1. Orbits
   2. Zygomatic arches
   3. Sinuses

(A) 1 only

(B) 1 and 3 only

(C) 2 and 3 only

(D) 1, 2, and 3

32. Which cranial bone articulates with all of the other cranial bones?

(A) Ethmoid

(B) Sphenoid

(C) Frontal

(D) Occipital

33. For the axiolateral projection (Schuller) of the temporomandibular joints, the skull is placed in a true lateral position and the central ray is directed

(A) 10° caudad.

(B) 10° cephalad.

(C) 30° caudad.

(D) 30° cephalad.

34. For the axiolateral oblique projection of the mandible, with the head in a true lateral position, the central ray is angled

(A) 10° cephalad.

(B) 10° caudad.

(C) 25° cephalad.

(D) 25° caudad.

Refer to the following image for Questions 35 and 36:

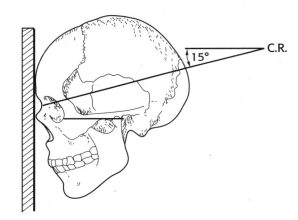

15° C.R.

35. The position being demonstrated in the figure above is which of the following methods?

(A) Caldwell

(B) Haas

(C) Towne

(D) Waters

GO ON TO THE NEXT PAGE ⟩

36. If the position of the skull stays the same, as in the figure above, but the central ray is directed perpendicular to the image receptor to exit the nasion, which bone will be BEST visualized?

    (A) Frontal

    (B) Sphenoid

    (C) Ethmoid

    (D) Occipital

37. The ankle mortise is demonstrated with which rotation?

    (A) 15° internal rotation

    (B) 15° external rotation

    (C) 45° internal rotation

    (D) 45° external rotation

38. The proximal tibiofibular articulation is seen as open with which projection of the knee?

    (A) AP

    (B) AP oblique, medial rotation

    (C) AP oblique, lateral rotation

    (D) Lateral

Refer to the following radiograph for Questions 39 to 41:

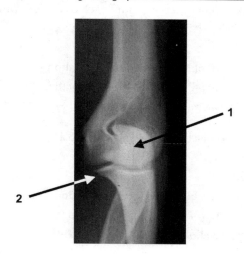

39. What projection of the elbow is seen in the radiograph above?

    (A) AP

    (B) AP oblique, internal rotation

    (C) AP oblique, external rotation

    (D) Lateral

40. Arrow 1 identifies the

    (A) radial head.

    (B) olecranon process.

    (C) capitulum.

    (D) trochlea.

41. Arrow 2 identifies the

    (A) radial head.

    (B) olecranon process.

    (C) coronoid process.

    (D) trochlea.

GO ON TO THE NEXT PAGE

KAPLAN)

42. The femoral epicondyles are placed perpendicular to the image receptor for which of the following projections of the knee?

    (A) AP

    (B) AP oblique knee, medial rotation

    (C) AP oblique knee, external rotation

    (D) Lateral

43. The projection of the ankle that places the calcaneus in profile is the

    (A) AP.

    (B) AP oblique, 45° medial rotation.

    (C) AP oblique, 15° medial rotation.

    (D) mediolateral.

44. For proper positioning, it is necessary to have the shoulder, elbow, and wrist in the same horizontal plane for which of the following projections?

    1. AP forearm
    2. Lateral elbow
    3. PA hand

    (A) 1 only

    (B) 1 and 2 only

    (C) 2 and 3 only

    (D) 1, 2, and 3

45. What is the degree of rotation for oblique projections of the wrist?

    (A) 10°

    (B) 20°

    (C) 45°

    (D) 60°

46. Which radiographic study requires the use of a radiolucent ruler within the image to measure differences in limb lengths?

    (A) Bone survey

    (B) Long bone measurement

    (C) Bone age

    (D) Soft-tissue study

47. If patient condition allows, the foot should be dorsiflexed for which of the following projections?

    1. AP ankle
    2. Lateral ankle
    3. Axial calcaneus

    (A) 1 only

    (B) 1 and 2 only

    (C) 2 and 3 only

    (D) 1, 2, and 3

Refer to the following image for Question 48:

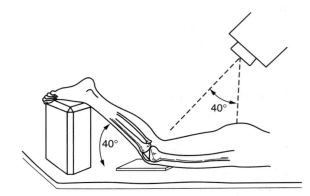

48. The patient position demonstrated in the figure above is the

    (A) PA knee.

    (B) PA axial, intercondylar fossa.

    (C) PA patella.

    (D) tangential patella.

49. The centering point for an AP axial projection of the toes is the

    (A) third distal interphalangeal joint.

    (B) third proximal interphalangeal joint.

    (C) third metatarsophalangeal joint.

    (D) third cuneiform.

GO ON TO THE NEXT PAGE ▷

50. For an AP projection of the scapula, the arm should be

    (A) internally rotated.

    (B) abducted 90° from the body.

    (C) adducted to the body.

    (D) neutral.

51. Which structure is located between the greater and lesser tubercle of the humerus?

    (A) Bicipital groove

    (B) Anatomical neck

    (C) Surgical neck

    (D) Body

52. The base of the fifth metatarsal is best demonstrated with which projection of the foot?

    (A) AP

    (B) AP oblique, medial rotation

    (C) AP oblique, lateral rotation

    (D) AP axial

53. What is the proper centering point for an AP thumb?

    (A) PIP

    (B) DIP

    (C) Interphalangeal joint

    (D) MCP

Refer to the following radiograph for Questions 54 to 56:

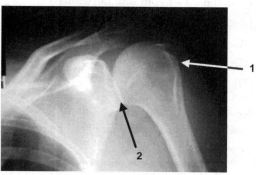

© DxR Development Group, Inc.

54. The radiograph above indicates which projection of the shoulder?

    (A) AP oblique (Grashey)

    (B) AP, neutral

    (C) AP, internal rotation

    (D) AP, external rotation

55. Arrow 1 identifies which structure?

    (A) Greater tubercle

    (B) Lesser tubercle

    (C) Coracoid process

    (D) Acromion process

56. Arrow 2 identifies which articulation?

    (A) Sternoclavicular

    (B) Acromioclavicular

    (C) Scapulohumeral

    (D) Humeroradial

GO ON TO THE NEXT PAGE

57. Which movement of the wrist best demonstrates the scaphoid without foreshortening?

(A) External rotation

(B) Internal rotation

(C) Radial deviation

(D) Ulnar deviation

58. For which view of the elbow will the humeral epicondyles appear superimposed on the radiograph?

(A) AP

(B) AP, medial oblique

(C) AP, lateral oblique

(D) Lateral

59. Which of the following procedures could be performed to evaluate the ligaments surrounding a joint?

(A) Venography

(B) Arthrography

(C) Lymphography

(D) Myelography

60. Which of the following procedures could be performed to rule out a deep vein thrombosis of the lower extremity?

(A) Angiography

(B) Venography

(C) Arthrography

(D) Lymphography

61. An AP thoracic spine examination is performed using the following technique: 20 mAs, 80 kVp, 60" SID. If the kVp is reduced to 68 and the SID is decreased to 45", how will the image be affected?

(A) Increased detail and decreased contrast

(B) Increased detail and increased contrast

(C) Decreased detail and increased contrast

(D) Decreased detail and decreased contrast

62. The humidity in the radiographic film storage area should not exceed

(A) 40 percent.

(B) 50 percent.

(C) 60 percent.

(D) 70 percent.

63. Films that have a brownish appearance that appears months or weeks after the examination are probably the result of

(A) inadequate developer retention.

(B) inadequate fixer retention.

(C) increased developer retention.

(D) increased fixer retention.

Refer to the following radiograph for Question 64:

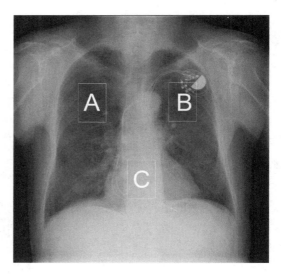

64. Which ionization chamber(s) should be selected for a chest examination on the patient pictured above?

(A) A

(B) B

(C) C

(D) A and C

GO ON TO THE NEXT PAGE

65. Compared to film-screen systems, photostimulable phosphor (PSP) plates used in computed radiography demonstrate

    (A) wider exposure latitude and lower spatial resolution.

    (B) wider exposure latitude and greater spatial resolution.

    (C) narrower exposure latitude and greater spatial resolution.

    (D) narrower exposure latitude and lower spatial resolution.

66. Which of the following intensifying screen phosphor is NOT currently in use today?

    (A) Gadolinium

    (B) Yttrium

    (C) Calcium tungstate

    (D) Lanthanum

67. Which of the following changes will result in a radiographic image with increased radiographic contrast?

    (A) Increasing the SID from 40" to 48"

    (B) Decreasing the grid ratio from 12:1 to 8:1

    (C) Increasing the screen speed from 200 to 400

    (D) Collimating from a 12"'×"'12 field size to a 5 × 5 field size

68. Which of the following will occur if automatic processor chemicals are under-replenished?

    1. Decreased contrast
    2. Decreased detail
    3. Decreased density

    (A) 1 and 2 only

    (B) 1 and 3 only

    (C) 2 and 3 only

    (D) 1, 2, and 3

69. The primary purpose of the intensifying screen is to

    (A) reduce patient dose.

    (B) increase contrast.

    (C) increase detail.

    (D) protect the film.

Refer to the following radiograph for Question 70:

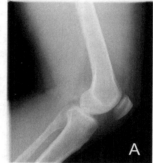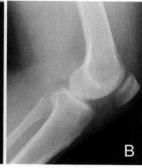

70. Which of the following statements could be true of images A and B displayed above?

    1. Image A was performed with a larger SID if OID was the same.
    2. Image A was performed with a larger OID if SID was the same.
    3. Image A displays increased recorded detail.

    (A) 1 and 2 only

    (B) 1 and 3 only

    (C) 2 and 3 only

    (D) 1, 2, and 3

71. A technique chart used for automatic exposure control systems will list all factors needed to produce a radiograph EXCEPT which of the following?

    (A) mA

    (B) Time

    (C) kVp

    (D) SID

GO ON TO THE NEXT PAGE

KAPLAN

72. Which of the following general conditions would require an increase in radiographic technique in order to produce an appropriate radiographic density?

    (A) Elderly patient
    (B) Emaciated patient
    (C) Atrophied musculature
    (D) Heavy musculature

73. Which of the following cast types would require an increase in technical factors to maintain radiographic density?

    (A) Recently placed fiberglass cast
    (B) Dry fiberglass cast
    (C) Pneumatic splint
    (D) Dry plaster cast

74. An AP ankle radiograph is performed on a pediatric patient in the emergency department using 5 mAs, 70 kVp, a 40" SID, and a small focal spot. Upon review, it is determined that the image needs to be repeated in order to increase radiographic density. Which change listed below would increase radiographic density without altering the image in any other way?

    (A) Increase the kVp to 80
    (B) Increase the mAs to 10
    (C) Decrease the SID to 36"
    (D) Utilize a large focal spot

Refer to the following image for Question 75:

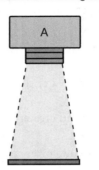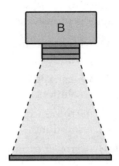

75. Which of the following statements is true of the two tube/image receptor situations displayed above?

    (A) Setup A would result in a greater demonstration of the heel effect.
    (B) Setup B would result in a greater demonstration of the heel effect.
    (C) Setup B would result in increased recorded detail.
    (D) Setup A would result in increased recorded detail.

76. An image is produced using a 5:1 grid and 25 mAs. If the image is repeated using a 12:1 grid, what new mAs setting will be required in order to maintain radiographic density?

    (A) 10
    (B) 29
    (C) 50
    (D) 63

GO ON TO THE NEXT PAGE ▷

77. An image is performed using a 40" SID, a 12" OID, a small focal spot size, and a 200-speed screen. Which of the following changes will increase the size distortion seen on the completed image?

    1. Decrease the SID to 36"
    2. Increase the screen speed to 400
    3. Increase the OID to 15"

    (A) 1 and 2 only
    (B) 1 and 3 only
    (C) 2 and 3 only
    (D) 1, 2, and 3

78. Although it is good practice to include this on a completed image, which of the following pieces of information is not required to be attached to every radiographic image?

    (A) Patient identifier
    (B) Technologist identifier
    (C) Date of examination
    (D) Right or left marker

79. The transport system of an automatic processor consists of a drive motor, gear assembly, roller assembly, and

    (A) recirculation pumps.
    (B) holding tanks.
    (C) cross-over racks.
    (D) air tubes.

Refer to the following image for Question 80:

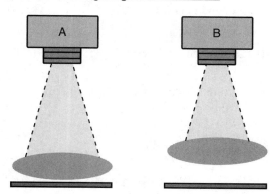

80. If two images were performed using the same technical factors and the tube-patient-image receptor setups displayed above, Setup B would result in increased

    (A) contrast.
    (B) detail.
    (C) density.
    (D) noise.

81. At the start of the workday, a film is processed in an automatic processor before the processor has had time to properly warm up. The resulting film will display

    (A) increased density and increased contrast.
    (B) increased density and decreased contrast.
    (C) decreased density and decreased contrast.
    (D) decreased density and increased contrast.

82. Which of the following would be considered voluntary motion?

    (A) Tremors
    (B) Peristalsis
    (C) Heartbeat
    (D) Breathing

GO ON TO THE NEXT PAGE

KAPLAN

83. How does poor film-screen contact appear on a finished radiograph?

(A) An overall light film

(B) A film with light areas

(C) A film with areas of blur

(D) A film with blur across the entire film

84. Which of the following statements is TRUE regarding an automatic processor?

(A) Development chemicals should never get into the fixer tank.

(B) The water coming into the processor is from the cold water supply line.

(C) "Starter" must be added to the developer tank every day.

(D) Damp films are always the result of a malfunction in the dryer.

Refer to the following radiographs for Question 85:

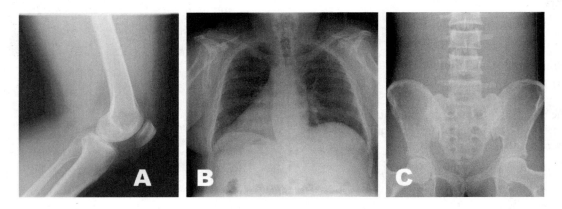

85. Which image shown above displays the greatest amount of subject contrast?

(A) A

(B) B

(C) C

(D) All images display the same amount.

GO ON TO THE NEXT PAGE

86. Which type of imaging system is capable of providing the quickest image display?

    (A) Photostimulable phosphor plates

    (B) Direct digital solid-state detectors

    (C) Film/screen using automatic processing

    (D) Film/screen using manual processing

87. Increasing kVp without making any other change to radiographic technique will

    (A) increase density and increase contrast.

    (B) increase density and decrease contrast.

    (C) decrease density and decrease contrast.

    (D) decrease density and increase contrast.

88. Which of the following changes will increase recorded detail?

    1. Decreasing the RPM of anode rotation
    2. Decreasing the angle of the anode
    3. Decreasing the size of the actual focal spot

    (A) 1 and 2 only

    (B) 1 and 3 only

    (C) 2 and 3 only

    (D) 1, 2, and 3

89. Increasing film-screen speed without making any other changes to radiographic technique will

    (A) increase density and increase detail.

    (B) increase density and decrease detail.

    (C) decrease density and decrease detail.

    (D) decrease density and increase detail.

90. Film that is stored in an environment that is too high in temperature is more likely to exhibit

    (A) increased density.

    (B) increased contrast.

    (C) decreased detail.

    (D) pressure marks.

Refer to the following radiograph for Question 91:

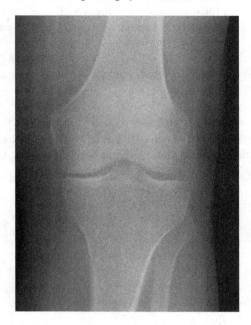

91. What is the name given to the artifact seen on the above radiograph?

    (A) Motion

    (B) Noise

    (C) Elongation

    (D) Foreshortening

92. An AP cervical spine radiograph is performed at 12 mAs and a 40" SID. If the exam is repeated at a 50" SID, what should the new mAs setting be in order to maintain radiographic density?

    (A) 14

    (B) 15

    (C) 19

    (D) 24

GO ON TO THE NEXT PAGE

KAPLAN

93. This device is used to measure how easily light can travel through a radiographic film. It is often used daily to verify the status of an automatic processor.

    (A) Densitometer
    (B) Sensitometer
    (C) Pentrometer
    (D) Photometer

94. What is a quick and straightforward way of determining if a digital image has been overexposed?

    (A) Analyze the image to determine if it is too dark
    (B) View the image to determine if the contrast is too low
    (C) Compare exposure indicators with manufacturer standards
    (D) Look for noise across the entire image

Refer to the following radiograph for Question 95:

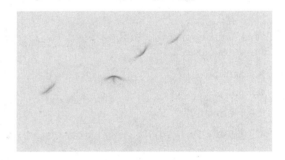

95. The artifacts shown above are caused by

    (A) dirt in the cassette.
    (B) rough handling.
    (C) a scratched screen.
    (D) a processor malfunction.

96. An individual "box" of visual information used to create a digital image that varies in density from white to black is called a

    (A) pixel.
    (B) matrix.
    (C) bit.
    (D) byte.

97. An image is performed with a beam filtration of 2.5 mm Al/Eq. If the filtration is increased to 3 mm Al/Eq and the examination is repeated, the second image will display

    (A) increased density.
    (B) decreased detail.
    (C) decreased contrast.
    (D) increased magnification.

98. An image is performed with a 50" SID. The resulting image is too light and it is decided that distance will be used adjust radiographic density. By adjusting the SID to 25", radiographic density will

    (A) increase by a factor of 2.
    (B) increase by a factor of 4.
    (C) decrease by a factor of 4.
    (D) decrease by a factor of 2.

99. A PA chest radiograph is performed on two patients, each with a 2 inch tumor located just under the scapula. One patient's body habitus is asthenic and the other's is hypersthenic. When compared to the asthenic patient, the tumor of the hypersthenic patient will appear

    (A) larger with increased detail.
    (B) larger with decreased detail.
    (C) smaller with decreased detail.
    (D) smaller with increased detail.

GO ON TO THE NEXT PAGE

Refer to the following image for Question 100:

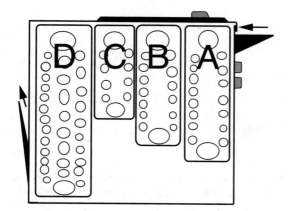

100. In the illustration above, in which section of an automatic processor will the latent image first become visible?

(A) A

(B) B

(C) C

(D) D

101. "Minus densities" can be caused by which of the following?

1. Roller pick-off
2. Screen scratches
3. Dirt in a cassette

(A) 1 and 2 only

(B) 1 and 3 only

(C) 2 and 3 only

(D) 1, 2, and 3

102. Which one of the following techniques would produce the highest radiographic contrast?

(A) 50 mAs, 75 kVp, 40" SID, 8:1 grid, 100-speed screen, small focal spot

(B) 200 mAs, 64 kVp, 44" SID, 12:1 grid, 100-speed screen, small focal spot

(C) 100 mAs, 87 kVp, 40" SID, 12:1 grid, 200-speed screen, large focal spot

(D) 400 mAs, 100 kVp, 48" SID, 6:1 grid, 100-speed screen, large focal spot

103. What are the primary purposes of a PACS system?

1. Storage of digital images
2. Distribution of images
3. Digital image processing

(A) 1 and 2 only

(B) 1 and 3 only

(C) 2 and 3 only

(D) 1, 2, and 3

104. Which of the following events will most significantly decrease recorded detail?

(A) Changing the OID from 3" to 4"

(B) Allowing a patient to move 1 inch during the exposure

(C) Using a 400-speed intensifying screen instead of a 200-speed intensifying screen

(D) Using a large focal spot size rather than a small focal spot size

GO ON TO THE NEXT PAGE

KAPLAN

Refer to the following radiograph for Question 105:

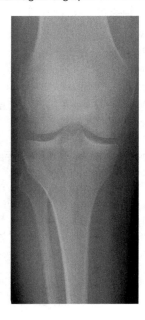

105. The image displayed above demonstrates

 (A) foreshortening.

 (B) grid cutoff.

 (C) elongation.

 (D) motion.

106. Which of the following statements is true regarding fixed and variable kVp technique chart systems?

 (A) Fixed kVp systems utilize the same kVp for all exams.

 (B) Fixed kVp systems result in generally higher patient dose than variable kVp systems.

 (C) Variable kVp systems provide better contrast than fixed kVp systems.

 (D) Variable kVp systems are not able to make small changes in radiographic exposure.

107. When additional filtration is added to the X-ray beam,

 (A) technical factors should be increased to compensate.

 (B) technical factors should be decreased to compensate.

 (C) no adjustment should be made to technical factors.

 (D) no exposure should be made because this can damage the tube.

108. Which of the following statements is true regarding double versus single film-screen systems?

 (A) Double film-screen systems exhibit increased speed and increased detail.

 (B) Double film-screen systems exhibit decreased speed and increased detail.

 (C) Double film-screen systems exhibit decreased speed and decreased detail.

 (D) Double film-screen systems exhibit increased speed and decreased detail.

109. In order to reduce shape distortion, the central ray should be directed

 (A) perpendicular to the anatomical part and perpendicular to the image receptor.

 (B) perpendicular to the anatomical part and parallel to the image receptor.

 (C) parallel to the anatomical part and perpendicular to the image receptor.

 (D) parallel to the anatomical part and parallel to the image receptor.

GO ON TO THE NEXT PAGE

Refer to the following diagram for Question 110:

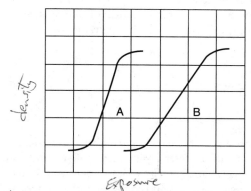

110. If the same technical factors are used to expose the two films displayed on the D log E curves displayed above, Film A will display

(A) increased density and increased contrast.

(B) increased density and decreased contrast.

(C) decreased density and decreased contrast.

(D) decreased density and increased contrast.

111. According to radiation safety standards, which of the following are characteristics of the fluoroscopy exposure switch?

1. It should be a 6-foot-long cord.
2. It should be a dead-man type.
3. It should terminate fluoroscopy after 5 minutes.

(A) 1 only

(B) 2 only

(C) 2 and 3 only

(D) 1, 2, and 3

112. The process that reduces exposure to the patient's skin by absorbing low-energy photons from a heterogeneous beam and "hardening" the beam is called

(A) collimation.

(B) filtration.

(C) positive beam limitation (PBL).

(D) total filtration.

113. A patient who has undergone radiation therapy for breast cancer presents with vomiting, diarrhea, and lethargy. Laboratory studies reveal a reduced number of lymphocytes, erythrocytes, and platelets. It is determined that she was exposed to a radiation dose of 250 rad. This exposure can lead to

(A) central nervous system syndrome.

(B) hematologic syndrome.

(C) gastrointestinal syndrome.

(D) renal syndrome.

114. A 24-year-old woman has a routine chest X-ray performed. Three days later she returns and informs staff that she is pregnant. Which of the following is the most appropriate action that should be taken by the radiologic technologist?

(A) Inform the supervising radiographer and the hospital's medical ethics committee

(B) Inform the radiologist and advise the patient that fetal exposure should be measured

(C) Perform a fetal ultrasound

(D) Reassure the patient and send her home

GO ON TO THE NEXT PAGE

KAPLAN

115. Institutions use dosimetry services to process film badges and other types of dosimeters to prepare personnel monitoring reports. Which of the following are included in the report?

    1. Image quality
    2. Personal data
    3. Type of dosimeter

(A) 1 only

(B) 2 only

(C) 2 and 3 only

(D) 1, 2, and 3

116. Jane Doe, a 26-year-old female who is three months pregnant, arrives at the hospital with her elderly mother, who is unable to stand for an X-ray. Which of the following individuals should hold the elderly patient during the procedure?

(A) Jane Doe

(B) Mammographer

(C) Nurse

(D) Radiologic technologist

117. Late effects of radiation are not observed for months or years. Which of the following is a late effect of radiation?

(A) Central nervous system syndrome

(B) Cytogenic damage

(C) Hematologic depression

(D) Leukemia

118. Which of the following techniques should be employed to reduce the effects of patient motion in pediatric radiography?

    1. Low mA station
    2. Proper immobilization techniques
    3. Short exposure times

(A) 1 only

(B) 1 and 2 only

(C) 2 and 3 only

(D) 1, 2, and 3

119. If a reaction is produced by 5 Gy of a test radiation and it takes 25 Gy of 250 kVp X-rays to produce the same reaction, what is the relative biologic effectiveness of the test radiation?

(A) 0.20

(B) 4

(C) 5

(D) 20

120. According to the inverse square law, if a radiographer stands 2 meters away from an X-ray tube, she will receive an exposure of 4 mR per hour. What will the exposure be if the radiographer moves 4 meters from the X-ray tube?

(A) 1 R

(B) 1 mR

(C) 2 mR

(D) 0.5 mR

121. A radiologic technologist who works in a cardiac catheterization unit is determining which dosimeter to use. Which personal dosimeter is a self-reading device that can provide an immediate readout for workers in high-exposure areas?

(A) Densitometer

(B) Film badge

(C) Pocket ionization chamber

(D) Thermal luminescent dosimeter

122. Which of the following factors does not affect the amount of exposure received by a patient?

(A) Collimation

(B) Filtration

(C) OID

(D) SID

GO ON TO THE NEXT PAGE

123. Which of the following is the portion of the cell cycle that is the period of cellular growth between divisions?

(A) Anaphase

(B) Interphase

(C) Prophase

(D) Telophase

124. Which of the following methods should the radiographer utilize to decrease the patient's voluntary motion?

1. Shortening the exposure time while increasing milliamperes (mA)
2. Utilizing high-speed imaging receptors
3. Gaining the cooperation of the patient

(A) 1 only

(B) 2 only

(C) 3 only

(D) 1, 2, and 3

125. Which of the following cells is LEAST radiosensitive?

(A) Endothelial cell

(B) Intestinal crypt cell

(C) Nerve cells

(D) Spermatids

126. Which of the following acts as an X-ray beam limitation device to reduce the amount of scatter radiation?

(A) X-ray tube

(B) Collimator

(C) Film

(D) Anode focal spot

127. Which of the following cause tissue damage by the production of free radicals?

1. Alpha particles
2. Gamma rays
3. X-rays

(A) 1 only

(B) 2 only

(C) 1 and 2 only

(D) 2 and 3 only

128. During a barium enema, which of the following factors will reduce the amount of patient dose?

1. Exposure switch
2. Source-to-skin distance
3. X-ray intensity

(A) 1 only

(B) 2 only

(C) 3 only

(D) 1, 2, and 3

129. Which dosimeter is light-free and contains a crystalline form of lithium fluoride as its sensing material?

(A) Film badge

(B) Optically stimulated luminescent dosimeter

(C) Pocket ionizing chambers

(D) Thermal luminescent dosimeter

130. An exposure was taken at 50 mAs, 70 kVp and 40" SID. What factors must a radiographer use in order to reduce the patient dose and maintain the same density?

(A) 50 mAs, 80 kVp, 40" SID

(B) 25 mAs, 80 kVp, 40" SID

(C) 60 mAs, 60 kVp, 48" SID

(D) 50 mAs, 70 kVp, 72" SID

GO ON TO THE NEXT PAGE

KAPLAN

131. According to local and federal requirements, the ionization chamber and the electrometer system should be calibrated for evaluation of which of the following?

1. Half-value layer
2. Reproducibility of output
3. Tabletop exposure rates for fluoroscopic units

(A) 1 only
(B) 2 only
(C) 1 and 2 only
(D) 1, 2, and 3

132. Which of the following is a late somatic effect of radiation?

1. Cataractogenesis
2. Embryologic defects
3. Erythema

(A) 1 only
(B) 2 only
(C) 1 and 2 only
(D) 1, 2, and 3

133. While taking a mobile radiograph, which of the following increases patient dose?

(A) Adequate source-skin distance of at least 12 inches (30 cm)
(B) Proper collimation and shielding
(C) Radiographic grid
(D) Using high kVp and low mAs

134. Which of following structural shields is located perpendicular to the primary X-ray beam?

1. Primary protective barrier
2. Secondary protective barrier
3. Control booth barrier

(A) 1 only
(B) 2 only
(C) 1 and 2 only
(D) 1, 2, and 3

135. According to the Target theory, which of the following organelles should be inactivated for cell death to occur?

(A) Endoplasmic reticulum
(B) Golgi apparatus
(C) Mitochondria
(D) Nucleus

136. Which of the following factors should be taken into account by the radiographer when attaining a mobile radiographic image?

1. Distance from the primary beam
2. Shielding
3. Position of the radiographer   90° angle of beam

(A) 1 only
(B) 2 only
(C) 1 and 2 only
(D) 1, 2, and 3

137. A 15-year-old female comes into the hospital with a complaint of persistent cough. The referring physician orders AP and Lateral chest films to rule out pneumonia. What factors must be used to reduce radiation exposure to the patient?

1. Gonadal shielding devices
2. Proper collimation of the X-ray beam
3. Use of a flat contact shield

(A) 1 only
(B) 1 and 2 only
(C) 2 and 3 only
(D) 1, 2, and 3

138. Which types of radiation should be accounted for when designing an X-ray room?

1. Leakage radiation
2. Primary radiation
3. Scatter radiation

(A) 1 only
(B) 2 only
(C) 1 and 2 only
(D) 1, 2, and 3

GO ON TO THE NEXT PAGE

KAPLAN

139. If an exposure produces 10 mrem at 1 second, what would the exposure be if the time was reduced to 0.50 seconds?

(A) 5.0 mrem

(B) 5.5 mrem

(C) 7.0 mrem

(D) 20 mrem

140. Which of the following are components of the film badge?

1. Assorted metal filters
2. Durable, lightweight plastic film holder
3. Film packet

(A) 1 only

(B) 2 only

(C) 1 and 2 only

(D) 1, 2, and 3

141. Which of the following measures should be taken while obtaining a mobile X-ray?

1. The radiographer should be 6 feet away from both the patient and the X-ray tube.
2. The radiographer must announce that an exposure is about to be made, and wait for personnel and visitors to leave the area.
3. The SID should be kept as low as possible.

(A) 1 only

(B) 2 only

(C) 1 and 2 only

(D) 1, 2, and 3

142. A nuclear medicine facility was contaminated by radioactive material. Which type of gas-filled radiation survey instrument should be used to monitor the facility?

(A) Dosimeter

(B) Geiger-Müller (G-M) detector

(C) Ionization chamber-type survey meter (cutie pie)

(D) Proportional counter

Refer to the following diagram for Question 143:

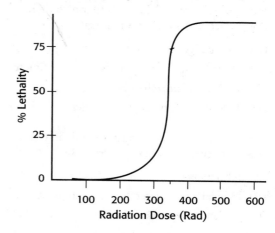

143. Referring to the diagram above, which of the following is the estimated radiation dose that will produce 75 percent lethality in humans within 30 days?

(A) 100 rad

(B) 300 rad

(C) 350 rad

(D) 400 rad

144. Fluoroscopy and special procedures produce the highest occupational exposure to health care workers. During a procedure, where should the dosimeter be worn?

(A) At collar level over the lead apron

(B) On the sleeve

(C) Underneath the lead apron

(D) None of the above

145. Which of the following modalities are likely to produce the highest occupational dose?

1. Diagnostic radiography
2. Magnification radiography
3. Mammography

(A) 1 only

(B) 2 only

(C) 3 only

(D) 1, 2, and 3

GO ON TO THE NEXT PAGE

KAPLAN

146. Of the four types of personnel dosimeters used to measure exposure of the body to ionizing radiation, which is the most economical?

    (A) Film badge
    (B) Optically stimulated luminescent dosimeter
    (C) Pocket ionizing chambers
    (D) Thermal luminescent dosimeter

147. Which dosimeter is the most accurate in terms of assessing entrance skin exposure (ESE)?

    (A) Film badge
    (B) Optically stimulated luminescent dosimeter
    (C) Pocket ionizing chambers
    (D) Thermal luminescent dosimeter

148. A mammographer leaves her film badge on a park bench during a humid summer afternoon. Which of the following results would be expected from the dosimetry film?

    (A) An accurate reading
    (B) Falsely high readings
    (C) Falsely low readings
    (D) None of the above

149. Interaction with free-radical species is a result of which of the following phenomena?

    (A) Apoptosis
    (B) Direct action
    (C) Indirect action
    (D) None of the above

150. Filtration is a reduction of low-energy beams that cause scatter. During an exposure above 70 kVp, how much filtration should be used?

    (A) 0.5 mm aluminum equivalent
    (B) 1.0 mm aluminum equivalent
    (C) 1.5 mm aluminum equivalent
    (D) 2.5 mm aluminum equivalent

151. The cascading effect that occurs from electrons of an outer shell filling the hole in an inner shell that occurs in target atoms and generates X-ray photon emission occurs during the

    (A) Compton effect.
    (B) photoelectric effect.
    (C) characteristic effect.
    (D) bremmstrahlung effect.

152. Where in the X-ray circuit is kilovoltage first generated?

    (A) Primary side of the autotransformer
    (B) Secondary side of the autotransformer
    (C) Primary side of the step-up transformer
    (D) Secondary side of the step-up transformer

153. The deceleration of electrons at the X-ray tube target results in what percentage of X-ray production?

    (A) 100%
    (B) 99%
    (C) 25%
    (D) 1%

154. In the diagnostic X-ray range, which of the interactions of radiation with matter is determined by the cube of the energy and the cube of the atomic number of the material irradiated?

    (A) Classical scattering
    (B) Compton effect
    (C) Photoelectric effect
    (D) Pair production

155. In the development of a positron during pair production, if the energy of the incident photon is 7.5 MeV, the energy of the positron would be

    (A) 1.02 MeV.
    (B) 3.75 MeV.
    (C) 0.51 MeV.
    (D) 3.24 MeV.

GO ON TO THE NEXT PAGE

156. Which of the following tests should be performed to check for appropriate film/screen contact?

    (A) Nine-penny test
    (B) Wire mesh test
    (C) Spinning top test
    (D) Phantom testing

157. Which of the following meters or measuring devices is the most appropriate instrument for checking the accuracy of the timer in a three-phase full wave rectified X-ray unit?

    (A) Oscilloscope
    (B) Penetrometer
    (C) Densitometer
    (D) Sensitometer

158. An optical density (OD) reading of 3.0 indicates that _____ percent of light was transmitted to the area being measured from a radiographic image.

    (A) 10 percent
    (B) 1 percent
    (C) 0.1 percent
    (D) 0.01 percent

159. Which of the following materials may be used in the construction of the X-ray tube target?

    1. Tungsten
    2. Molybdenum
    3. Lead

    (A) 1 only
    (B) 1 and 3 only
    (C) 1 and 2 only
    (D) 1, 2, and 3

160. The range of diagnostic tube target angles is

    (A) 1–5°.
    (B) 7–17°.
    (C) 15–25°.
    (D) 30–40°.

161. Which of the following types of units could be referred to as a dedicated X-ray unit?

    1. Panorex
    2. Mammography
    3. General radiographic

    (A) 1 only
    (B) 1 and 2 only
    (C) 2 and 3 only
    (D) 1, 2, and 3

162. The rotor of the X-ray tube, which allows the anode to spin, is made to turn by the power of a(n)

    (A) induction motor.
    (B) transformer.
    (C) direct current motor.
    (D) rectifier.

163. For electromagnetic mutual induction to work correctly in a transformer, the primary coil must be supplied with a(n)

    (A) pulsating direct current.
    (B) direct current.
    (C) alternating current.
    (D) pulsating alternating current.

164. The positively charged electrode of the X-ray tube is called the

    (A) glass envelope.
    (B) X-ray window.
    (C) anode.
    (D) cathode.

GO ON TO THE NEXT PAGE

KAPLAN

165. Which of the following characteristics is not true of X-ray photons?

    (A) They are electrically neutral.
    (B) They release very large amounts of heat upon passing through matter.
    (C) They travel at the speed of light.
    (D) They produce secondary and scatter radiation.

166. Which of the following electrical devices will read the electromotive force (EMF) in an electrical circuit?

    (A) Densitometer
    (B) Circuit breaker
    (C) Ammeter
    (D) Voltmeter

167. When utilizing automatic exposure control devices (AECs), the backup timer cannot exceed what percentage of the anticipated manual exposure mAs?

    (A) 50%
    (B) 100%
    (C) 150%
    (D) 200%

168. Using automatic exposure control devices and abiding by U.S. Public Law 90-602, generators must terminate exposures at what mAs for exposures above 50 kVp?

    (A) 100 mAs
    (B) 200 mAs
    (C) 400 mAs
    (D) 600 mAs

169. Photoelectric effect is dependent upon the energy of the incident photon as well as the atomic number of the material imaged. Photoelectric effect occurs more readily in bone than in oxygenated tissue since the atomic number of oxygen is 8 while the atomic number of bone, or calcium, is

    (A) 13.
    (B) 20.
    (C) 50.
    (D) 56.

170. Regarding atomic structure, the term atomic number refers to the number of _____ contained in an atom.

    (A) electrons
    (B) protons
    (C) electron shells
    (D) neutrons

171. Variations between the stated kilovoltage and the X-ray beam quality must be within what percentage of the desired kilovoltage setting?

    (A) ± 1%
    (B) ± 2%
    (C) ± 5%
    (D) ± 10%

172. The type of graph used to represent the acceptable range of optical density in processed radiographic images is known as a(n)

    (A) linear, dose-response curve.
    (B) nonlinear, dose-response curve.
    (C) sensitometric curve.
    (D) anode cooling curve.

GO ON TO THE NEXT PAGE

173. When performing a radiographic exam, the image is primarily created by what type of interaction?

    (A) Compton scatter
    (B) Coherent scatter
    (C) Photoelectric absorption
    (D) Photodisintegration

174. What process ensures that electrons flow only from the cathode to the anode in the X-ray tube?

    (A) Mutual induction
    (B) Self induction
    (C) Line compensation
    (D) Rectification

175. Which of the following legal documents would list the decision of the patient should he become unable to communicate his instructions at a time of terminal illness or permanent unconsciousness?

    (A) DNR
    (B) DRG
    (C) Living will
    (D) Medical records

176. *Res ipsa loquitur* translates as

    (A) quid pro quo.
    (B) this for that.
    (C) the master speaks for the servant.
    (D) the thing speaks for itself.

177. Which of the following items must be included in the Introduction of Contrast Material and Radiopharmaceuticals Data Sheet?

    1. Patient allergies
    2. Time of administration
    3. Name of the individual who administered the contrast material

    (A) 1 only
    (B) 2 only
    (C) 1 and 3 only
    (D) 1, 2, and 3

178. The ethical principle that places high value on avoiding doing harm to others is called

    (A) nonmaleficence.
    (B) fidelity.
    (C) morals.
    (D) autonomy.

179. The consent that allows for an unconscious patient, as in the case of severe head injury, permission to undergo procedures relevant to care is called

    (A) emergency.
    (B) informed.
    (C) valid.
    (D) implied.

180. A deaf patient will rely most on which type of communication?

    (A) Demonstration
    (B) Verbal
    (C) Palpation
    (D) Simple vocabulary

181. When interviewing a patient, which of the following would be considered good questioning skills?

    (A) Asking open-ended questions
    (B) Using silence
    (C) Using repetition
    (D) All of the above

182. The effective use of oral communication would include

    (A) giving clear instructions that the patient understands.
    (B) using proper pronunciation.
    (C) speaking clearly.
    (D) All of the above

GO ON TO THE NEXT PAGE

183. Hand-washing is a form of

   (A) medical asepsis.

   (B) surgical asepsis.

   (D) disinfection.

   (C) sterilization.

184. Which of the following is the most common method used to sterilize small medical equipment?

   (A) Chemical

   (B) Dry heat

   (C) Autoclaving

   (D) Gas plasma

185. Standard precautions designed to reduce the transmission of bloodborne and pathogenic agents apply to all of the following EXCEPT

   (A) blood.

   (B) sweat.

   (C) mucous membranes.

   (D) all body fluids.

186. The exterior assembly of a urinary drainage device must always remain in which position?

   (A) On the table next to the patient

   (B) Level with patient's bladder

   (C) Higher than the patient's bladder

   (D) Lower than the patient's bladder

187. When opening a sterile procedure tray for a radiographic procedure containing sterile instruments, which flap of the sterile package will be opened first?

   (A) The flap opened to the right

   (B) The flap opened to the left

   (C) The flap opened away from the radiographer

   (D) The flap opened toward the radiographer

188. Which of the following special precautions would the radiographer take when entering the isolation room of a patient who has tuberculosis?

   (A) Wear a particulate air filter respirator mask

   (B) Wear a gown upon entering the patient room

   (C) Wash hands before entering the room and wear gloves

   (D) All of the above

189. The correct number of room air changes per hour for a patient with measles, placed in an isolation room, is

   (A) 1 to 2.

   (B) 6 to 12.

   (C) 12 to 20.

   (D) 20 to 40.

190. Which of the following is considered a bacterial infection?

   (A) Strep throat

   (B) AIDS

   (C) Herpes simplex

   (D) Hepatitis

Refer to the following illustration for Question 191:

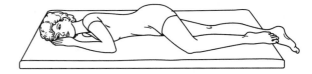

191. Which type of patient position is demonstrated above?

   (A) Trendelenburg

   (B) Fowler's

   (C) Prone

   (D) Sims'

GO ON TO THE NEXT PAGE

192. For a two-person lift transfer, the wheelchair should be placed facing the X-ray table at what angle?

    (A) 45° to the table

    (B) 90° to the table

    (C) 180° to the table

    (D) Parallel to the table

Refer to the following graph for Question 193:

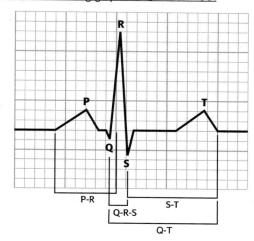

193. On the ECG tracing above, the QRS complex represents the

    (A) contraction of the atria.

    (B) contraction of the ventricles.

    (C) relaxation of the atria.

    (D) relaxation of the ventricles.

194. The medical term that means "shortness of breath" is

    (A) cyanosis.

    (B) bradypnea.

    (C) dyspnea.

    (D) hypoxia.

195. When performing an intramuscular injection, the needle should be inserted into the muscle at an angle of

    (A) 90°.

    (B) 45°.

    (C) 30°.

    (D) 15°.

196. Normal adult BUN blood lab values are between

    (A) 7 and 18 mg/dL.

    (B) 15 and 250 mg/dL.

    (C) 0.6 and 1.7 mg/dL.

    (D) 1.6 and 7.0 mg/dL.

197. Barium is what type of contrast agent?

    (A) Negative

    (B) Positive

    (C) Neutral

    (D) Specialty

198. Of the reactions listed below, which type of reaction to a contrast media injection would not be considered mild?

    (A) Hypotension

    (B) Metallic taste

    (C) Urticaria

    (D) Vomiting

GO ON TO THE NEXT PAGE

KAPLAN

Refer to the following image for Questions 199 and 200:

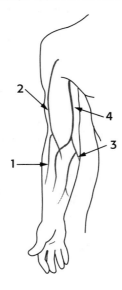

199. In the figure above, the vein identified by Number 1 is the

   (A) cephalic.
   (B) accessory cephalic.
   (C) antecubital.
   (D) basilic.

200. The vein identified by Number 4 is the

   (a) cephalic.
   (b) accessory cephalic.
   (c) antecubital.
   (d) basilic.

Practice Test Answers and Explanations

1. The correct answer is (A).

The only articulations between the upper limbs and the trunk are the sternoclavicular joints. They are formed by the articulation between the sternal extremity of the clavicles and the clavicular notches of the manubrium. These joints are synovial, gliding joints that permit free movement.

2. The correct answer is (B).

Determining air-fluid levels (pleural effusion) requires a completely horizontal central ray, as in an erect or decubitus chest position. If the chest image is taken with the patient in a supine or semierect position, the pleural effusion will obscure vascular lung markings when compared with a fully erect chest projection.

3. The correct answer is (B).

The proximal esophagus (3) is located posterior to the trachea (4), and continues down through the mediastinum anterior to the descending aorta (2) until it passes through the diaphragm into the stomach. The heart (1) is located in the very anterior aspect of the thoracic cavity, directly behind the sternum.

4. The correct answer is (D).

The AP lordotic projection, demonstrated here, is performed primarily to rule out calcifications and masses beneath the clavicles, especially in the area of the apices and upper lungs.

5. The correct answer is (A).

For the true lateral position of the chest, the coronal plane is perpendicular and the sagittal plane is parallel to the plane of the image receptor; the central ray is directed to midthorax at the level of T7 (3 to 4" below the level of the jugular notch).

6. The correct answer is (B).

When using the body rotation method for sternoclavicular joints, position the patient on enough of an oblique angle to project the vertebrae well behind the joint closest to the IR. The angle is usually about 10 to 15°. So for visualization of the left sternoclavicular joint, the patient should be in a 10 to 15°, LAO position.

7. The correct answer is (C).

Hirschsprung disease is a congenital condition of the large intestine in which the neurons controlling rhythmic contractions are missing. Atresia (A) is a congenital condition where an opening to an organ is absent; surgery is required. In celiac disease (B), a congenital condition as well, certain protein found in wheat causes an allergic reaction in the intestinal lining. Volvulus (D) is a mechanical obstruction caused by a twisting of the intestine itself.

8. The correct answer is (B).

The prone position is used to compress the abdominal contents, which increases radiographic quality. For the final radiographs of thin patients, it may be necessary to angle the table into the Trendelenburg position (C) to unfold superimposed loops of the ileum.

9. The correct answer is (C).

For the AP projection during an upper GI series, on a sthenic type of patient, the central ray and IR are centered to the level of L1 (midway between the xiphoid tip and the lower margin of the ribs). For the hypersthenic patient, the central ray is directed 1 inch above L1; for the asthenic patient, the central ray is directed 2 inches below L1.

10. The correct answer is (B).

The small bowel series requires that radiographs be done at timed intervals. The oral ingestion of barium is preceded by a preliminary radiograph of the abdomen (scout). Each radiograph of the small intestine is identified with a time marker indicating the interval between the exposure and the initial ingestion of barium.

11. The correct answer is (A).

The liver (Arrow 1) is the organ that forms bile. The gland secretes bile at the rate of 1 to 3 pints each day. The gallbladder (Arrow 4) stores the bile temporarily. The duodenum (Arrow 3) is the first portion of the small intestine.

12. The correct answer is (B).

The two main hepatic ducts emerge to form the common hepatic duct, which in turn unites with the cystic duct to form the common bile duct. The common bile duct joins the pancreatic duct, and together they enter the ampulla of Vater (hepatopancreatic ampulla). The ampulla of Vater then opens into the descending portion of the duodenum.

13. The correct answer is (C).

The pancreas is both an exocrine and endocrine gland. The exocrine cells produce pancreatic juice, which acts on proteins, fats, and carbohydrates. The endocrine portion (consisting of islet cells, or islets of Langerhans) produces hormones insulin and glucagons, which are responsible for sugar metabolism.

14. The correct answer is (B).

To demonstrate small amounts of intraperitoneal gas in acute abdominal cases, the patient should remain on her left side for optimally 10 to 20 minutes, or at least 5 minutes, before obtaining the left lateral decubitus image. In this position, the air rises to an area under the right hemidiaphragm, where it will not be superimposed by the gastric bubble (liver used as contrast to the air). If the patient is unable to lie on her left side, right lateral decubitus can be performed.

15. The correct answer is (D).

The body habitus greatly affects the location of organs within the abdominal cavity. Sthenic is the average body build. Hypersthenic (B), the most massive body build, is about 5 percent of the population. Hyposthenic/asthenic individuals are more slender and have narrow and longer lungs; they also usually have a lower diaphragm and stomach.

16. The correct answer is (A).

The renal calyces appear as hollowed, flattened tubes. From 4 to 13 minor calyces (Arrow 1) unite to form 2 to 3 major calyces.

17. The correct answer is (D).

The ureter is identified by Arrow 4. The renal parenchyma (Arrow 2) is a general term used to describe the total functional portions of the kidneys, such as those visualized during an early phase of an intravenous urogram procedure. The renal pelvis (Arrow 3) is formed by the uniting of the major calyces and each expanded renal pelvis narrows to continue as the ureter (Arrow 4).

18. The correct answer is (B).

For IVU, one should review the patient's clinical history, allergic history, and blood chemistry levels. The normal creatinine level is 0.6 to 1.5 mg/100 mL, and the normal BUN (blood urea nitrogen) level is 8 to 25 mg/100 mL. Any levels elevated higher than that suggest renal dysfunction and should be reviewed by a physician before any procedure is started.

19. The correct answer is (B).

The AP erect position, post-void, demonstrates nephroptosis (positional change of the kidneys).

20. The correct answer is (C).

For an AP pelvis, center the central ray and image receptor midway between the ASIS and the pubic symphysis (approximately 2 inches inferior to the ASIS and 2 inches superior to the pubic symphysis in an average-sized patient).

21. The correct answer is (A).

Anklyosing spondylitis (Marie Strümpell disease) is a progressive form of arthritis; it mainly involves the spine, and joints and articulations—especially the sacroiliac joints—become ankylosed (fused). Herniated nucleus pulposus (HNP) (B) is a herniation of the nucleus pulposus of the disk through a rupture in the annulus fibrosus. Spina bifida (C) is an anomaly characterized by incomplete closure of the vertebral canal. Scoliosis (D) is an abnormal lateral curvature of the spine.

22. The correct answer is (B).

Lateral swimmers will help demonstrate a lateral projection of the lower cervical and upper thoracic vertebrae between the two shoulders.

23. The correct answer is (C).

Using the Judd method for a PA projection of the dens and atlas as seen through the foramen magnum, the patient is in the prone position; the patient extends the neck to rest the chin until the OML forms a 37° angle to the plane of the image receptor (chin and mastoid tip are perpendicular).

24. The correct answer is (D).

The Judd or Fuchs method for demonstrating the upper portion of the odontoid should not be performed if the patient has degenerative disease, unhealed fracture, or suspected fracture of the upper cervical region (perhaps the patient is wearing a cervical collar).

25. The correct answer is (A).

A typical cervical vertebra (C3–C6) has a small, oblong body. The transverse processes arise partly from the sides of the body and partly from the vertebral arch. These processes are short and wide, and are perforated by transverse foramina (Arrow 4) for the transmission of the vertebral artery and vein. The spinous processes (Arrow 1) have short bifid tips.

26. The correct answer is (B).

The superior and inferior articular facets form the zygapophyseal joints in the articulated vertebral column. The superior and inferior articular processes are located posterior to the transverse processes at the point where the pedicles and laminae unite.

27. The correct answer is (D).

When a patient arrives at the emergency department with traumatic injury, one of the first assessments done by the physician is an evaluation of the spine. A cross-table lateral cervical projection, used to detect up to 90 percent of significant injuries, should be performed first and cleared by a physician before moving the patient or removing any cervical collar.

28. The correct answer is (C).

For the AP axial, L5–S1 projection of the lumbar spine the central ray is angled 30° for male patients and 35° for female patients, ~~caudad~~. Radiographs may also be obtained prone, but with a caudal angle.   *cephalic*

29. The correct answer is (B).

The AP or PA axial projection with the 30 to 35° central ray angulation to 2″ superior to the pubic symphysis results in an image that shows the lumbosacral joint and symmetric image of both sacroiliac joints free of superimposition.

30. The correct answer is (D).

The parietoacanthial projection (Waters) projects the petrous ridges below the maxillary sinuses.

31. The correct answer is (D).

The parietoacanthial projection (Waters) can be utilized for all of the following: orbits, zygomatic arches, and sinuses. (It can also be used for nasal bones, facial bones, and a modification for the mandible.)

32. The correct answer is (B).

The sphenoid bone articulates with each of the other seven bones of the cranium.

33. The correct answer is (C).

The head is adjusted into a true lateral position and the central ray is angled 25 to 30° caudad, centered to 0.5" anterior and 2" superior to upside EAM. The TMJ nearest the image receptor is visible. The closed-mouth image demonstrates the condyle within the mandibular fossa; the condyle moves to the anterior margin of the fossa in the open-mouth position.

34. The correct answer is (C).

For the axiolateral projection of the mandible, place the head in a true lateral position for demonstration of the ramus. The central ray is directed 25° cephalad, slightly inferior and posterior to the gonion farthest from the image receptor.

35. The correct answer is (A).

The positioning described in the figure is the PA axial, Caldwell method. The central ray is angled 15° caudad to exit the nasion.

36. The correct answer is (A).

For a PA projection of the cranium, place the OML perpendicular to the plane of the image receptor. If the frontal bone is of primary interest, direct the central ray perpendicular to exit the nasion.

37. The correct answer is (A).

The ankle joint is often called the ankle mortise or mortise joint. It is formed by the articulations between the lateral malleolus of the fibula and the inferior surface and medial malleolus of the tibia. To demonstrate the ankle mortise, the entire leg and foot together are rotated internally 15 to 20° until the intermalleolar plane is parallel with the image receptor.

38. The correct answer is (B).

The AP oblique medial rotation of 45° demonstrates the proximal tibiofibular joint and the head of the fibula.

39. The correct answer is (B).

The AP oblique internal rotation demonstrates the coronoid process of the ulna in profile, and the olecranon process within the olecranon fossa.

40. The correct answer is (B).

The AP oblique projection, medial rotation, demonstrates the olecranon process (Arrow 1) seated in the olecranon fossa.

KAPLAN

41. The correct answer is (C).

A correct 45° internal rotation visualizes the coronoid process of the ulna in profile (Arrow 2).

42. The correct answer is (D).

The femoral epicondyles are directly superimposed and the plane of the patella is perpendicular to the plane of the image receptor for a lateral projection of the knee. The femoral epicondyles are parallel with the image receptor for a true AP projection of the knee.

43. The correct answer is (D).

The lateral projection of the ankle (mediolateral or lateromedial) places the calcaneus in lateral profile.

44. The correct answer is (B).

For all projections of the forearm, elbow, and wrist, it is necessary to seat the patient at the end of the table with the elbow flexed about 90° and the hand and wrist resting on the cassette, palm down. Drop the patient's shoulder so that the shoulder, elbow, and wrist are on the same horizontal plane. For projections of the hand, the same applies, except it is not necessary to have the shoulder, elbow, and wrist on the same horizontal plane.

45. The correct answer is (C).

For the PA oblique, lateral rotation, and the AP oblique, medial rotation, projections of the wrist, the part is rotated 45°. For the PA oblique, lateral rotation, projection, the scaphoid and trapezium are well demonstrated; for the AP oblique, internal rotation, the pisiform is seen as separate from the adjacent carpal bones.

46. The correct answer is (B).

Accurate measurements of the length of long bones—specifically length differences between the two sides—can be evaluated through long bone measurement. Although studies are occasionally made of the upper limbs, radiography is most frequently applied to the lower limbs. For lower extremities, a metal measurement ruler is placed between the patient's lower limbs and three exposures are made at the joints of the hips, knees, and ankles.

47. The correct answer is (D).

The foot is dorsiflexed, when possible, for all views of the leg, ankle, calcaneus, and lateral foot projection.

48. The correct answer is (B).

The PA axial projection (Camp-Coventry) demonstrates an unobstructed projection of the intercondyloid fossa and the medial and lateral intercondylar tubercles of the intercondylar eminence.

49. The correct answer is (C).

For the AP axial projection of the toes, the central ray is directed 15° through the third metatar-sophalangeal joint (MTP). The image demonstrates the 14 phalanges of the toes and the distal portions of the metatarsals and the interphalangeal joints.

50. The correct answer is (B).

For an AP projection of the scapula, the patient is asked to abduct the arm to a right angle with the body to draw the scapula laterally.

51. The correct answer is (A).

The lesser tubercle is situated on the anterior surface of the humerus, immediately below the anatomic neck (B). The greater tubercle is located on the lateral surface of the humerus, just below the anatomic neck, and is separated from the lesser tubercle by a deep depression called the intertubercular (bicipital) groove.

52. The correct answer is (A). *B*

The AP oblique, medial rotation, demonstrates the third through fifth metatarsals free of superim-position. The tuberosity at the base of the fifth metatarsal is seen in profile and well visualized.

53. The correct answer is (D).

For an AP thumb, the hand is internally rotated until the posterior surface of the thumb is in contact with the image receptor; the central ray is directed to the first metacarpophalangeal joint (MCP). There is no distal and proximal interphalangeal joint of the thumb—only one inter-phalangeal joint.

54. The correct answer is (D).

The AP external rotation of the shoulder places the greater tubercle and humeral head in profile.

55. The correct answer is (A).

The greater tubercle is located on the lateral portion of the proximal humerus just below the ana-tomic neck. It is seen in profile with the AP, external rotation, projection.

56. The correct answer is (C).

The scapulohumeral articulation between the glenoid cavity and the head of the humerus forms a synovial ball-and-socket joint, allowing movement in all directions.

57. The correct answer is (D).

The PA projection, with ulnar deviation, best demonstrates the scaphoid with adjacent articula-tions open.

58. The correct answer is (D).

The lateral projection of the elbow demonstrates the elbow joint, distal arm, and proximal forearm. The humeral epicondyles are superimposed.

59. The correct answer is (B).

Arthrography is a contrast-media study of synovial joints and their related soft tissue. The hip, knee, ankle, elbow, shoulder, and TMJs are common for arthrography. Venography (A) is the study of veins, lymphography (C) is performed to visualize the lymph vessels and nerves, and myelography (D) visualizes the spinal canal.

60. The correct answer is (B).

Lower-limb venography is common and is usually performed to rule out thrombosis of the deep veins of the leg.

61. The correct answer is (C).

kVp is the primary controller of contrast; as kVp decreases, contrast increases, due to the reduction in the production of scatter radiation. SID greatly affects radiographic detail by affecting both geometric fuzzinesss and size distortion; as SID increases, detail decreases. In this question, the kVp decreases (contrast increases) and SID decreases (detail decreases).

62. The correct answer is (C).

High humidity in an area where film is stored can cause condensation to collect on film. Humidity that is too low (below 30 percent) may lead to static artifacts.

63. The correct answer is (D).

When the fixing agent is not properly removed from the film emulsion in the wash, it continues to work and slowly oxidizes the emulsion, which leads to a brownish appearance. The fixing agent is sometimes referred to as *hypo*, so the term "hypo retention" is often used to describe increased fixer retention.

64. The correct answer is (A).

The presence of a pacemaker presents a positioning challenge for a radiographer if automatic exposure control (AEC) is utilized. If Chamber B was selected, it is possible that the examination would result in overexposure because the X-ray photons would attempt to penetrate the pacemaker prior to terminating the exposure. Chamber C presents the same problem because it too will result in an image with a density higher than optimal.

65. The correct answer is (A).

PSP plates used in computed radiography demonstrate a much wider exposure latitude than film-screen systems. In other words, PSP plates are able to compensate for low or high exposures and display an image of diagnostic quality. If high or low exposures are used with film-screen imaging systems, the films will be too dark or too light. Film-screen systems do produce greater spatial resolution (detail), but the ability to manipulate exposure data in a computed radiography system are seen by many as a great advantage in imaging.

66. The correct answer is (C).

Calcium tungstate was commonly used as an intensifying screen material until the 1970s when new phosphor types were established. These phosphors, which contain gadolinium, yttrium, and lanthanum, are able to provide the same image quality as calcium tungstate screens at approximately 25 percent of the radiographic dose requirement. Collectively, screens made from gadolinium, yttrium, and lanthanum are known as rare-earth screens.

67. The correct answer is (D).

Increasing collimation (collimating to a smaller field size) improves contrast because less tissue is radiated and therefore less scattered radiation is produced. Collimation also helps to reduce patient dose because it reduces the amount of tissue that is exposed to ionizing radiation. SID and screen speed have virtually no effect on contrast. Grids do affect contrast, but a change from a lower-ratio grid to a higher-ratio grid (from 5:1 to 10:1, for example) is necessary to increase radiographic contrast.

68. The correct answer is (B).

The proper balance of chemistry in an automatic processor is critical to producing a quality image. When chemistry is under-replenished, the chemicals are weaker than what is necessary and the quality of the film degrades. The chemicals in an under-replenished processor are not able to produce a desired density, nor is there a capacity for the processor to create appropriate contrast on the finished film. Although the resultant film will look "ugly" due to the poor contrast and density, detail is not directly affected by the processor; detail is determined by exposure factors such as screen speed, focal spot size, and SID.

69. The correct answer is (A).

The reason screens exist at all is to reduce the amount of radiation needed to create an image and thus reduce the dose to the patient. Consider an AP lumbar spine radiograph produced at 50 mAs with a 300-speed screen. If the screen were removed, the technique would have to be increased to 7,500 mAs in order to maintain density! Although screens do decrease detail as compared to direct exposure, the savings in dose more than compensates for the change. Screens do slightly increase contrast when changing from a direct exposure to a screen technique, and intensifying screen cassettes do protect the film, but these are not primary purposes of the intensifying screens or cassettes.

70. The correct answer is (B).

SID and OID greatly affect the recorded detail seen on a completed radiographic image. As SID increases, detail increases and magnification decreases. Because Image A is the least magnified of the two images, it must be the one performed at the larger SID. A film that was performed with a larger OID would demonstrate increased magnification and decreased detail.

71. The correct answer is (B).

Automatic exposure control (AEC) regulates the time setting for an exposure and therefore does not appear on a technique chart. All other factors should appear on a technique chart used for AEC in order to ensure consistent image quality.

72. The correct answer is (D).

Because muscle is slightly harder to penetrate than fatty tissue, patients who have well-developed musculature will require an increase in technical factors in order to produce a radiograph with appropriate density. The other conditions listed would require a decrease in technique in order to maintain density.

73. The correct answer is (D).

A dry plaster cast will require an increase in technique in order to properly penetrate the cast and display the underlying anatomy. A wet plaster cast will require an even greater increase. Fiberglass casts require no additional increase in technique beyond the technique that results from measuring the cast and setting an appropriate technique. Pneumatic splints are air-filled plastic splints that are very easy to penetrate.

74. The correct answer is (B).

mAs is the primary controller of radiographic density and should be the factor to change if a modification in density is desired. Radiographic density will not be affected if the small or large focal spot is used. The other two factors changed in this question, kVp and SID, will affect density but will also decrease the quality of the image. When kVp is increased, contrast will decrease; and when SID is decreased, detail will also decrease.

75. The correct answer is (B).

The heel effect is demonstrated to a greater extent whenever the collimator is open wide. In this case a larger film size is used in Setup B, so the result would be a greater demonstration of the heel effect. Using a short SID also leads to a greater opening of the collimator and increased demonstration of the heel effect; however, in this example, both setups use the same SID so detail would be the same for both images.

76. The correct answer is (D).

In order to solve this problem, the radiographer must first know the Bucky factors (grid factors). The average grid factors are as follows:

No Grid	1
5:1 Grid	2
8:1 Grid	4
12:1 Grid	5
16:1 Grid	6

Using these grid factors and the original mAs, use the following formula to find the new mAs.

$$\frac{mAs_1}{mAs_2} = \frac{Bucky\ factor_1}{Bucky\ factor_2}$$

$$\frac{25}{mAs_2} = \frac{2}{5}$$

Now solve for the new mAs by cross-multiplying and dividing by the original Bucky factor:

$$mAs_2 = 125/2$$

$$mAs_2 = 63$$

77. The correct answer is (B).

Size distortion is the misrepresentation of the size of an object by magnification. SID and OID determine the degree of magnification. As OID increases and/or SID decreases, magnification will increase. The degree of magnification can also affect detail in much the same way (as OID increases and/or SID decreases, detail will decrease), and screen speed can also affect detail (as screen speed increases, detail will decrease), but screen speed will not affect the magnification of an object.

78. The correct answer is (B).

Four pieces of information need to be listed on every radiographic image. Three of the four pieces are listed here, with the fourth being the facility at which the procedure was performed. Other pieces of information (including the technologist's initials, for example) are good practices but are not necessarily requirements.

79. The correct answer is (C).

Crossover racks, or "guideshoes," steer the film from one processing tank to the next as it is moved by the roller assembly. The recirculation pump and holding tanks are part of the recirculation system. Air tubes force hot air across the film and are found in the dryer.

80. The correct answer is (A).

Setup B is an illustration of the air-gap technique, an alternative to the use of a grid. Because of the increased OID, less scattered radiation strikes the image receptor and contrast is improved. Because the SID has not changed, the increased OID will also lead to decreased detail (B) and a slight decrease in density (C) due to the decreased number of scattered photons reaching the image receptor. Noise (D) is a result of decreased mAs; since the mAs did not change in this case, there will be no effect on noise.

81. The correct answer is (C).

An automatic processor is designed to be used with the chemical temperature adjusted to a specific setting. If the temperature is too low (such as using the processor before it has warmed up), the chemicals will not be able to perform as they were designed. This will lead to a decrease in density and a decrease in radiographic contrast.

KAPLAN

82. The correct answer is (D).

Breathing is a type of motion that can be controlled, even if it can be controlled for only a short time. Patients have no control over tremors, digestion (peristalsis), or cardiac function (heartbeat). To reduce the possibility of motion artifacts appearing on a radiographic image, proper patient communication techniques must be utilized.

83. The correct answer is (C).

Poor film-screen contact occurs whenever the film and screen fail to make sufficient contact. This may be caused by a warped cassette or by air, moisture, or dirt in between the screen and the film. This occurs in small areas of the cassette and not across the cassette as a whole (since the film and screen will have to make contact somewhere).

84. The correct answer is (B).

The temperature regulation system of the automatic processor uses heating elements to raise the water/chemical temperature to the desired level. If the incoming water is hot, the processor is not able to cool the water; therefore, it is very important that only cold water enters the processor. Development chemicals continuously enter the fixer tank (A) as the film leaves the development tank and enters the fixer tank. Starter (C) is used only when the processor has been cleaned and a brand-new batch of chemicals is used to fill the developer tank. Damp films (D) are most often the result of inadequate developer chemistry causing a "softening" of the radiographic film.

85. The correct image choice is (B).

Subject contrast refers to the amount of contrast present within the anatomical structures being examined. The greater the density difference between structures, the greater the subject contrast. In the case of the three images shown in this question, the chest radiograph has the greatest difference in densities; the ribs and spine are difficult to penetrate, whereas the air and lung tissue are easy to penetrate. The knee and lower abdomen radiographs display subject contrast as well because the bones, muscles, and organs differ in density, but the difference is not as great as that found in the anatomical area of the chest.

86. The correct answer is (B).

One of the primary advantages of using direct digital radiography systems is the speed with which the image becomes visible. Direct digital systems provide an almost instantaneous access to the radiographic image, whereas photostimulable phosphor plates must be physically carried to an analog/digital converter for processing. Film-screen processing requires even longer times because the film must be removed from the cassette and placed into either an automatic processor (requiring at least 90 seconds for processing) or processed by hand (taking up to 20 minutes just to complete the developing and fixing steps).

87. The correct answer is (B).

As kVp is increased, contrast decreases due to an increase in the production of scattered radiation. Density increases dramatically when kVp is increased, requiring only a 15 percent increase in kVp to effectively double the radiographic density on an image.

88. The correct answer is (C).

The effective focal spot is the most important contributing factor of the anode to radiographic detail. The effective focal spot is the measurable image of the area on the anode where X-rays are produced (the actual focal spot). The smaller the effective focal spot, the greater the recorded detail will be. Since the effective focal spot is dependent on the actual focal spot, the smaller the actual focal spot, the smaller the effective focal spot will be. The effective focal spot is also influenced by the angle of anode; the smaller the angle of the anode, the smaller the effective focal spot will be. The rotational speed of the anode does not affect the effective focal spot size; it is intended to protect the anode from thermal damage.

89. The correct answer is (B).

Film-screen speed refers to the speed at which a film will gain density. A film-screen combination with increased speed (a *fast* combination) will display increased density quicker than a film-screen combination with decreased speed (a *slow* combination). So using a fast combination will allow a radiographer to produce a radiograph with less exposure than what would be necessary with a slow combination, thereby decreasing the dose to the patient. The tradeoff for the increased speed is a reduction in recorded detail. As film-screen combinations increase, recorded detail decreases.

90. The correct answer is (A).

Stored film absorbs energy from heat and radiation while it sits on a shelf. If the filmed is stored for too long or is affected by excessive heat or scattered radiation, the film will demonstrate fog (increased density) on the finished film. This will also reduce contrast (B) but have no effect on detail (C).

91. The correct answer is (B).

Noise is the result of a low mAs technique. The mAs may be set abnormally low due to the use of very fast screens or a high kVp technique. In either case, not enough photons are produced to create an entire image and only a partial image is displayed.

92. The correct answer is (C).

The exposure maintenance formula (also known as the direct square law) must be used to solve this problem (New mAs = Old mAs × New Distance^2/Old Distance^2). In this case, New mAs = 12 × 2,500/1,600. If the 15 percent rule is utilized (used for increasing kVp), the result will be choice (A). If the exposure maintenance formula is used without squaring the distances, choice (B) will result. If the mAs is simply doubled, choice (D) will result. These are all common errors.

93. The correct answer is (A).

Sensitometry is the name of the process that tests the quality of the processing system. Ideally, sensitometry is performed daily to ensure that a processor is working correctly before patient images are developed. The process begins by placing a series of known exposures on a piece of film with a small machine called a *sensitometer* (B). The film is then processed and a densitometer is used to read the densities on the film. Even small variations in these readings can translate into noticeable changes on a processed film. A *pentrometer* (C) is a step wedge used to place a series of densities on a film through the use of an X-ray tube. A *photometer* (D) is used to measure light, such as the ambient light in a room or the brightness of a light box.

94. The correct answer is (C).

Exposure indicators (S-number, EI, log-mean, EXI) have been developed by digital imaging manufacturers to mathematically demonstrate the amount of radiation that has reached the image receptor. Because digital image processing is capable of adjusting density and contrast, it is difficult to determine overexposure by simply looking at a digital image. Noise occurs on a digital image when not enough X-ray photons have reached the image receptor to create a complete image (underexposure).

95. The correct answer is (B).

Rough handling of film in the darkroom caused the artifact displayed in this question. Whenever the film is bent, crescent marks like this will result.

96. The correct answer is (A).

Individual boxes of digitally displayed information are called pixels. Pixels may be white, black, or varying shades of gray. When enough pixels are put together, an image is formed. The matrix (B) is the name given to the number of pixels in a digital image. A bit (C) is the smallest unit of digital information, and a byte (D) is the name given to an 8-bit digital "word."

97. The correct answer is (C).

Filtration increases the average energy of the X-ray beam, effectively increasing kVp. Just as if kVp is increased, an increase in filtration will reduce contrast. Increasing filtration will also decrease radiographic density (A) but will not affect detail (B) or magnification (D).

98. The correct answer is (B).

Radiation intensity increases by the square of the change as distance decreases. In this case, distance was reduced by a factor of 2, so intensity will increase by a factor of 4 (or 2^2). The inverse square law can be used to illustrate this point further (an intensity of 100 mR is randomly assigned in this example):

$$\frac{\text{Original Intensity} \times}{\text{Original Distance}^2} = \frac{\text{New Intensity} \times \text{New}}{\text{Distance}^2}$$

$$100 \text{ mR} \times 50^2 = \text{New Intensity} \times 25^2$$

$$100 \text{ mR} \times 2{,}500 = \text{New Intensity} \times 625$$

$$250{,}000 = \text{New Intensity} \times 625$$

$$400 = \text{New Intensity}$$

Note that the intensity (and therefore the radiographic density) increased by a factor of 4.

99. The correct answer is (B).

A hypersthenic patient has a larger body habitus and therefore the tumor will be located farther from the image receptor during a PA chest examination. Due to the increased OID the tumor will also will be magnified more in the hypersthenic patient and will appear larger. The increase in OID due to the patient's body habitus also has an effect on the recorded detail of the image; increased OID leads to decreased recorded detail.

100. The correct answer is (A).

The developer is the first part of a processor that a film enters during the development process. It is in the developer that the latent image first becomes visible. If the film is pulled from the developer tank, the image will be visible; however, the development process will continue until the developed film is placed into the fixer tank (B), where development stops.

101. The correct answer is (D).

Minus densities are artifacts that appear white on a finished film. When rollers are dirty or sticky with residue, they will pick off or tear the emulsion from the film base. Minus densities will also occur if light from a screen is unable to reach the film due to scratches in the screen or dirt located between the screen and the film. Plus densities will appear dark and be caused by such things as poor film-screen contact, fog, or bending of the film.

102. The correct answer is (B).

In this list of radiographic techniques, the only factors that affect radiographic contrast are kVp and grids. Contrast improves as kVp decreases and grid ratio increases. The factors of mAs, SID, screen speed, and focal spot size can all be ignored when determining contrast. Choice (B) has the lowest kVp setting and utilizes the highest grid ratio; therefore, it produces the best contrast. Choice (D) produces the lowest contrast because it has the highest kVp setting and utilizes a 6:1 grid, which is the lowest of the choices in this question.

103. The correct answer is (A).

PACS stands for "picture archiving and communication system." Once the digital images have been processed during the acquisition stage of the digital imaging process, they are sent to the PACS. The PACS stores the images digitally and can be retrieved at any time by several users at the same time. The PACS is responsible for one of the greatest advantages of digital imaging over film-screen system, which is the ability of the PACS to distribute images to multiple locations at the same time, quickly and accurately.

104. The correct answer is (B).

Patient motion significantly reduces detail; even a small amount of motion can greatly reduce recorded detail. The other events listed in this question will all decrease recorded detail slightly, but moving 1 inch during the exposure will blur the anatomy of interest on the finished radiograph.

105. The correct answer is (C).

Elongation occurs when the X-ray tube or the image receptor is angled with respect to the anatomical part and creates an image that is longer than normal size. Foreshortening (A) occurs when the anatomical part is angled and the X-ray tube and image receptor are perpendicular to each other. This image was created with a tube angled along the long axis of the knee. Grid cutoff (B) can occur with angulation, but only when the tube is angled perpendicular to the grid lines. Motion (D) is identified by a blurring of the image; no motion is evident on this image.

106. The correct answer is (C).

In fixed kVp systems the kVp is set at the optimal kVp, which is the highest kVp setting that provides a quality radiographic image. This results in less overall dose to the patient but reduces contrast. The optimal kVp setting is fixed for various anatomical regions but does not vary in small increments like a variable kVp system.

107. The correct answer is (A).

Filters attenuate the X-ray beam just like a patient, the X-ray table, or a grid. Whenever something attenuates the beam, technical factors need to be increased to compensate.

108. The correct answer is (D).

Double film-screen systems consist of a film with two layers of emulsion, one on each side of the base, sandwiched between two intensifying screens. This configuration effectively doubles the speed of the double film-screen system. The tradeoff to increased speed is a decrease in recorded detail.

109. The correct answer is (A).

The least shape distortion occurs when the central ray is perpendicular to both the image receptor and the anatomical part. When the central ray is angled to both the anatomical part and the image receptor, elongation occurs. When the anatomical part is angled, foreshortening occurs.

110. The correct answer is (A).

The D log E curves displayed in this question provide a graphical representation of film speed and contrast. Film A displays increased speed because it is located to the right of Film B. The *x*-axis of the graph represents exposure and the *y*-axis represents density, so the D log E curves show that the same exposure will result in increased density on Film A. The steeper the curve, the higher the contrast provided by the film. Film A is steeper (more vertical) than Film B, so Film A displays increased contrast.

111. The correct answer is (B).

According to the radiation safety standard, the fluoroscopy exposure switch must be a dead-man type. Once the clinician's foot is released from the pedal, the exposure will automatically terminate. The 6-foot-long cord is associated with mobile radiography. The cumulative timer is an audible reminder that 5 minutes of fluoroscopy have been completed.

112. The correct answer is (B).

Essentially, filtration removes low-energy photons by absorbing them; subsequently, high-energy photons pass through the patient. This reduces patient dose. Collimation (A) is used to confine the X-ray beam. Positive beam limitation (PBL) (C) is a feature of the film cassette holder. It consists of electronic sensors that send signals to the collimator housing. This feature automatically adjusts the field size to match the film size. Total filtration (D) is the combination of added and inherent filtration.

113. The correct answer is (B).

The hematologic syndrome occurs after exposure to a radiation dose of 200 to 1,000 rad. An initial prodromal syndrome is followed by fever, vomiting, diarrhea, lethargy, and malaise. Laboratory studies will show a decrease in the number of lymphocytes, erythrocytes, and platelets. Keep in mind that all of these syndromes can present with vomiting, diarrhea, and lethargy. However, the hematologic changes and 250 rad exposure are distinguishing features.

In contrast, the central nervous system syndrome (A) occurs following radiation doses in excess of 5,000 rad. Adverse effects are acute and the patient may die in hours to days; initial symptoms of nausea and vomiting occur within minutes of the exposure. The syndrome progresses and the patient can experience disorientation, seizures, and coma. Death is often a result of increased intracranial pressure, vasculitis, or meningitis. The gastrointestinal syndrome (C) occurs following radiation doses of 1,000 to 5,000 rad. Prodromal vomiting and diarrhea are followed by anorexia, lethargy, and electrolyte imbalances. The renal syndrome (D) is not a known entity.

114. The correct answer is (B).

In cases that involve radiation and the unknowing pregnant patient, a radiologic physicist should be involved. In this way, fetal exposure can be determined. Fortunately, most cases will not result in significant damage to the fetus. Although protecting the fetus is of paramount importance, the physician may choose to have the pregnant patient undergo radiologic examination. This should be done if it is in the best interest of the patient. Remember, all females of child-bearing age should have a pregnancy test before a radiographic procedure.

KAPLAN

115. The correct answer is (C).

A personnel monitoring report should include the following: personal data, dosimeter type, quality of radiation, dose-equivalent data, and cumulative dose equivalents of each quarter year (3 months).

116. The correct answer is (C).

The preferred course of action in this situation is to use a mechanical restraint. In this case, because Jane Doe (A) is pregnant, she should not be exposed to radiation. However, friends or relatives that accompany the patient may be asked to help. Also, radiation employees such as the mammographer (B) and the radiologic technologist (D) should never be used to support patients. Finally, as a last resort, as is the case in this question, other health care workers (such as a nurse) may be asked to hold the patient.

117. The correct answer is (D).

The late effects of radiation include malignancies (including leukemia); local damage to the skin, gonads, and eyes; and shortened life span. These effects are not observed for months to years. On the other hand, early effects of radiation are observed minutes to days after the radiation exposure. Examples include cellular or cytogenetic damage (B); hematologic depression (C); local damage to the skin, gonads, or extremities; and acute radiation syndromes—including the central nervous system syndrome (A).

118. The correct answer is (C).

The technologist should take special care when working with the pediatric patient. It is important to note that children are more sensitive to the late somatic and genetic effects of radiation. The use of high mA station, immobilization techniques, and short exposure times will reduce the effects of patient motion in pediatric radiography.

119. The correct answer is (C).

The relative biologic effectiveness (RBE) is the relative capability of radiations with differing LETs to produce a particular biologic reaction. The RBE can be calculated as follows:

$$RBE = \frac{\text{Dose in Gy from 250 kVp X-rays}}{\text{Dose in Gy of test radiation}}$$

$$RBE = 25/5$$

$$RBE = 5$$

120. The correct answer is (B).

According to the inverse square law, "the intensity of radiation is inversely proportional to the square of the distance." In essence, as the distance from the X-ray tube increases, the intensity of the radiation decreases. The solution is as follows:

$$I_1 / I_2 = (D_2)^2/(D_1)^2$$
$$4 \text{ mR}/I_2 = (4 \text{ meters})^2/(2 \text{ meters})^2$$
$$I_2 = 1 \text{ mR}$$

121. The correct answer is (C).

A radiologic technologist who works in a high-exposure area such as a cardiac catheterization unit should use a pocket ionization chamber. These portable devices are highly sensitive, yet are infrequently used.

122. The correct answer is (C).

The object-to-image distance (OID) is a geometric factor that affects magnification and image detail. Collimation (A), filtration (B), and source-to-image distance (SID) (D) are factors used to reduce patient dose.

123. The correct answer is (B).

Interphase is the period of cellular growth between divisions. The phases of the cell cycle are: mitosis, G_1, S, and G_2. Mitosis is the phase of the cell cycle prophase (C); metaphase, anaphase (A), and telophase (D) are the phases of mitosis.

124. The correct answer is (C).

Voluntary motion can be eliminated by gaining the cooperation of the patient and immobilizing the patient during the exposure. Meanwhile, *involuntary motion* can be reduced by shortening exposure time and increasing milliamperes (mA) or utilizing high-speed imaging receptors.

125. The correct answer is (C).

Both nerve cells and muscle cells are among the least radiosensitive cell types. Endothelial cells (A), spermatids (D), osteoblasts, and fibroblasts have intermediate radiosensitivity. Highly radiosensitive cell types include erythroblasts, intestinal crypt cells (B), lymphocytes, and spermatogonia.

126. The correct answer is (B).

Collimators, aperture diaphragms, cones, and cylinders are used to limit X-ray beams and reduce scatter radiation.

127. The correct answer is (D).

Gamma rays and X-rays have a low linear energy transfer (LET). Low LET radiation can cause tissue damage via single-strand breaks or free-radical production. Fortunately, cellular damage caused by low LET radiation is usually reversible.

128. The correct answer is (B).

The source-to-skin distance should not be less than 38 cm on stationary fluoroscopes. Increasing the distance between the patient and the tube reduces patient dose. When the fluoroscopic tube is closer to the table top, the patient dose will be higher.

129. The correct answer is (D).

When lithium fluoride is irradiated, some electrons absorb energy, become "excited," and move to higher energy levels. When the device is heated, electrons move to an area known as the conduction band. The thermal luminescent dosimeter (TLD) analyzer determines the level of exposure to ionizing radiation. In effect, the amount of light emitted by the crystals is proportional to the TLD badge exposure.

Film badges (A) record whole-body radiation exposure. Internal filters measure the energy of the radiation that has reached the dosimeter. An optically stimulated luminescent dosimeter (B) can detect even low levels of X-ray and gamma photons. It is most useful for pregnant health care workers and those who work in low-radiation areas. Technologists who work in high-exposure areas, such as a cardiac catheterization unit, should use a pocket ionization chamber (C). These portable devices are highly sensitive, yet are infrequently used.

130. The correct answer is (B).

Increasing the kVp and decreasing mAs will reduce patient dose while maintaining the density. Increasing the distance (C and D) will reduce patient dose but will result in an underexposed radiograph. However, an increase in kVp along with an unchanged mAs and SID (A) will result in an overexposed film.

131. The correct answer is (D).

Both the ionization chamber and the electrometer system should be calibrated to evaluate the following factors: half-value layer, reproducibility of output, tabletop exposure rates for fluoroscopic units, and X-ray output in mR/mAs.

132. The correct answer is (C).

The late somatic effects of radiation include carcinogenesis, cataractogenesis, embryologic defects, and nonspecific life-span shortening. The early somatic effects of radiation include desquamation, epilation, erythema, fatigue, fever, gastrointestinal disturbances, nausea, and sterility.

133. The correct answer is (C).

In most cases, radiographic grids are used with mobile X-rays to improve radiographic contrast and detail. However, this results in increased patient dose. By increasing the source-to-skin distance (A), the radiographer can reduce the entrance exposure. Proper collimation and shielding (B), and the use of high kVp and low mAs (D), are proper methods of decreasing patient dose.

134. The correct answer is (A).

The role of a primary protective barrier is to impede primary radiation from affecting people on the other side of the barrier. The primary protective barrier is perpendicular to the direction of travel of the primary X-ray beam. A secondary protective barrier is located parallel to the X-ray beam; it overlaps the primary protective barrier. Control booth barriers serve to protect radiographers; they impede leakage and scatter radiation.

135. The correct answer is (D).

The key molecular "target" of radiation is DNA. Remember that cellular DNA is contained in the nucleus.

136. The correct answer is (D).

The radiographer should take account of all three factors while acquiring a mobile radiographic image. The distance from the primary beam allows the radiographer to use the inverse square law. Technologists must always wear protective garments (lead apron, gloves, thyroid shield) in order to shield themselves. Radiographers will receive the least amount of scatter radiation if they position themselves at a 90° angle from the beam.

137. The correct answer is (D).

Gonadal shielding should be used to protect the reproductive organs from exposure; it is a secondary protective measure. The different types of gonadal shielding include clear lead shielding, flat contact shields, shadow shields, and shaped contact shields. For females, using a flat contact shield over the reproductive organs reduces exposure by 50 percent. In addition, proper collimation is the primary method of reducing radiation exposure to the gonads.

138. The correct answer is (D).

Leakage radiation penetrates through the protective tube-housing and the sides of the collimator. Primary or direct radiation comes from the X-ray tube target. Scatter radiation is a result of Compton interactions; patients are the predominant source of such radiation.

139. The correct answer is (A).

Time and exposure are directly proportional, so reducing exposure time by half will reduce the exposure by 50 percent.

140. The correct answer is (D).

The film holder should be comprised of a low atomic number element to filter low energy X-radiation, gamma radiation, and beta radiation. Metal filters consist of aluminum and copper. The energy of the radiation that reaches the dosimeter is measured by these metal filters.

141. The correct answer is (C).

Mobile radiography is an area of high occupational exposure. Distance is the primary protective barrier when obtaining mobile films. Before the exam, a loud announcement should be made so family members, personnel, and other patients can leave the immediate area. The use of low source-to-image distance (SID) increases patient exposure and results in poor image detail.

142. The correct answer is (B).

This highly sensitive unit is able to detect electrons emitted from radioactive nuclei or photons. Therefore, it can detect any area contaminated by radioactive material. An audio alert will sound to indicate the presence of ionizing radiation. The G-M detector is the preferred tool for use in nuclear medicine facilities. The ionization chamber-type survey meter, or "cutie pie" (C), measures gamma and beta radiation. It is often used to measure exposure rates. Although the proportional counter (D) can distinguish between alpha and beta particles, it is not used in diagnostic radiography.

143. The correct answer is (C).

The $LD_{50/30}$ is defined as the dose of radiation that will cause death in half of the subjects within a time span of 30 days. It should be noted that the $LD_{50/30}$ for humans is 300 rad. In the diagram, draw a horizontal line from the y-axis until it intersects the S-curve, and then proceed vertically to the x-axis. The point at which the line intersects with the x-axis is $LD_{75/30}$. Therefore, in this example, the radiation dose is approximately 350 rad.

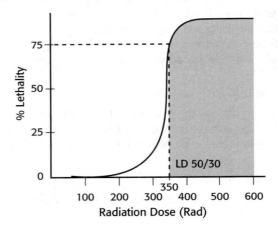

144. The correct answer is (A).

During fluoroscopy, the personal dosimeter should be worn at the collar level because the head, neck, and eyes receive 10 to 20 times more exposure than the body.

145. The correct answer is (A).

The highest personnel exposure is associated with diagnostic radiography, fluoroscopy, and portable X-ray procedures. Mammography uses low kVp exposure factors that produce very little scatter. Magnification radiography uses special equipment that utilizes small focal spots and increased OID.

146. The correct answer is (A).

The film badge is the most widely used and economical personnel dosimeter. It is lightweight and easy to carry.

147. The correct answer is (D).

The thermal luminescent dosimeter (TLD) is commonly used to measure skin dose. It determines the level of exposure to ionizing radiation. The amount of light emitted by the crystals is proportional to the TLD badge exposure. Film badges (A) record whole-body radiation exposure. Internal filters measure the energy of the radiation that has reached the dosimeter. An optically stimulated luminescent dosimeter (B) can detect even low levels of X-ray and gamma photons. It is most useful for pregnant health care workers and those who work in low-radiation areas. Pocket ionization chambers (C) are highly sensitive, portable devices that are used by technologists who work in high exposure areas, such as a cardiac catheterization unit.

148. The correct answer is (B).

If a film badge is exposed to sunlight for a prolonged period of time, the increasing temperature and humidity will cause falsely high readings.

149. The correct answer is (B).

The indirect action of free radicals on molecules such as DNA can result in biologic damage. On the contrary, if ionizing particles interact directly with DNA, enzymes, proteins, or RNA, it is known as direct action (C). Apoptosis (A) is programmed cell death that occurs as a result of the cellular effects of irradiation.

150. The correct answer is (D).

During an exposure above 70 kVp, a 2.5 mm aluminum equivalent is required. Similarly, for exposures that range from 50 to 70 kVP, a 1.5 mm aluminum equivalent should be used. Finally, in exposures below 50 kVp (mammography), a 0.5 mm aluminum equivalent should be utilized.

151. The correct answer is (C).

While Compton effect and photoelectric effect are interactions of radiation with matter, they occur within the human body, not at the X-ray tube target. Bremmstrahlung photons are created when they interact with the nuclear force field of target atoms.

152. The correct answer is (D).

Although the autotransformer is designated as the kV selector, it simply sets up the correct ratio of voltage that will be generated by the secondary side of the step-up transformer. The voltage sent to the primary side of the step-up transformer maintains the ratio of voltage to be converted to kilovoltage on the secondary side of the step-up transformer.

153. The correct answer is (D).

While the greatest amount of energy transformation is to thermal energy at 99 percent, only 1 percent of the energy transformation is for X-ray production.

154. The correct answer is (C).

Classical scattering occurs only with very low energy X-ray photons, and Compton effect is primarily based on the energy of the incident photon. As incident photon energy increases, the probability for Compton effect also increases. Pair production results in the development of two electrons and is used in nuclear medicine scanning for PET production.

155. The correct answer is (D).

In order to determine the resultant energy of the positron, you must subtract 1.02 from the initial energy and then divide by 2. In this example, $(7.5 - 1.02)/2 = 3.24$ would be the correct answer. The initial reaction requires an energy level of 1.02 MeV to create the positron and negatron; the remaining energy is equally transferred to the kinetic energy of the two particles.

156. The correct answer is (B).

The nine-penny test is used for light-field congruency; the spinning top test is to check for exposure times; and a phantom is a device used to mimic the attributes of human tissue.

157. The correct answer is (A).

The penetrometer is often referred to as a step wedge and gives a step-wedge appearance to a processed image. A sensitometer is a device designed to produce a reproducible uniform "step-wedge" image to a film, whereas a densitometer is a device that reads the optical density from a processed radiographic image.

158. The correct answer is (C).

Optical density (OD) measures the resultant darkness of an area in a radiographic image. The acceptable range for OD in an image is 0.25 to 2.5. The higher the OD number, the darker the area in the image. An OD number of 1 indicates that 10 percent of the light has been transmitted through that area on the image; an OD of 2 indicates 1 percent of the light was transmitted; and an OD of 4 indicates only 0.01 percent of the light has been transmitted through the image.

159. The correct answer is (C).

Lead is the material typically used for the tube enclosure of the X-ray tube. A common combination for the X-ray tube anode is tungsten, molybdenum, and rhenium, although molybdenum may be the specific target material in mammography tubes.

160. The correct answer is (B).

While a 12° angled anode is the most common, manufacturers do provide a range of anode angles to meet specific requirements when ordering an X-ray tube.

161. The correct answer is (B).

Dedicated X-ray units perform specific types of imaging procedures. While a panorex unit is used to image the mandible and dental area and a mammographic unit is used to image the breast, a general radiographic unit is utilized to image a variety of anatomical areas, such as the extremities and the abdomen.

162. The correct answer is (A).

A direct-current motor would not be effective in an X-ray tube because the tube operates on alternating current. Actually, an induction motor is a type of alternating-current motor. A transformer is used to regulate the voltage in a circuit, and a rectifier changes alternating equipment to pulsating direct current.

163. The correct answer is (C).

The flow of direct current is in one direction, which does not have the effect of continually cutting across the wires of the transformer as alternating current does. Alternating current continuously varies its direction every 1/120 of a second, so it sets up the changing magnetic fields across the primary and secondary sides of the transformer that are necessary for electromagnetic induction to occur. Because alternating current continuously changes direction, it is known as alternating current, not pulsating alternating current.

164. The correct answer is (C).

As with any electrical device, the positively charged portion (or electrode) is the anode, while the negatively charged portion is the cathode. The same is true for the terminals of a battery. The glass envelope is the specific enclosure around the electrodes of the X-ray tube that creates a vacuum around the electrodes, and the X-ray window is the thinner portion of the glass window through which the X-ray photons first pass once they are created.

165. The correct answer is (B).

If X-ray photons created high amounts of heat in matter, they would be potentially inappropriate for use in diagnostic imaging exams. The types of interactions that do occur with photons are cellular in nature and potentially do have other short-term and long-term risks to radiation exposure. X-ray photons do possess the other characteristics listed, such as being electrically neutral, traveling at the speed of light, and producing secondary and scatter radiations. In all, X-ray photons possess a total of 12 characteristics.

166. The correct answer is (D).

First, one must remember that the term *emf* is synonymous with voltage and potential difference; therefore, the instrument needed to read voltage would be a voltmeter. A densitometer reads the optical density (OD) in a radiographic image and an ammeter reads the current or number of electrons flowing through a circuit. A circuit breaker is a device used to monitor current flow through a circuit and will open if there is an overload in the circuit.

167. The correct answer is (C).

If an AEC were to allow only 50 percent or 100 percent of the anticipated manual mAs, then the resultant radiographic image might be too light, as with 50 percent, or properly exposed as with a 100 percent exposure length. Remember that the purpose of an AEC is to accommodate for varying patient thicknesses and pathologies, and so it needs the latitude to operate and compensate for these varying conditions. However, the ALARA concept is still important to maintain, so the highest backup exposure must be limited to 150 percent rather than 200 percent of the manual exposure.

168. The correct answer is (D).

The diagnostic imaging range extends from 23 to 150 kVp. For exposures below 50 kVp, such as for mammography, Public Law 90–602 allows for 2,000 mAs per exposure. For exposures above 50 kVp, where the majority of exposures are made, the maximum value of 600 mAs has been mandated. These limits allow for the use of contrast materials such as barium and the consideration for patient habitus and pathologies.

169. The correct answer is (B).

Consulting the periodic table of elements, one finds that 13 is the atomic number for aluminum, 50 is the atomic number for tin, and 56 is the atomic number for barium.

170. The correct answer is (B).

Atomic number may also be known as z number, and both refer to the number of protons in the nucleus of an atom. Mass number is the term used to describe the total number of protons and neutrons in the nucleus of an atom.

171. The correct answer is (C).

This means that if you have selected 70 kVp for a particular exposure, the actual peak usage of kilovoltage must be between 66.5 and 73.5 for the equipment to be in compliance. Determine this number by multiplying 70×0.05 (5 percent) to equal 3.5, and then subtract 3.5 from 70 to obtain the 66.5, or add 3.5 to 70 to obtain the 73.5 for this range.

172. The correct answer is (C).

Choices (A) and (B) both refer to curves used to predict biologic effects to ionizing radiation, such as stochastic or nonstochastic effects. Anode cooling curves are used to determine the safe operating capacity of the anode.

173. The correct answer is (C).

A radiographic image is created when some X-rays strike the image receptor while others are absorbed by anatomy within the body. Tissues with higher atomic numbers and greater densities (such as bone) absorb more radiation than fatty or muscular tissue; this difference in absorption translates into different densities on the image receptor. Photoelectric absorption is the type of interaction in which X-ray photons are absorbed.

174. The correct answer is (D).

Rectification refers to the changing of alternating current to pulsating direct current. Rectified current is very important to the operation of the X-ray tube by ensuring that electrons flow only from the cathode to the anode. If electrons are allowed to jump from the anode to the cathode, the cathode filament will be quickly destroyed and the tube will be rendered useless. Induction (A and B) refers to the electrical changes that occur in transformers. Line compensation (C) is the process of evening out the fluctuations of the incoming line voltage.

175. The correct answer is (C).

A living will is a legal document that lists the patient's decisions or instructions in case he is unable to communicate his wishes during terminal illness or permanent unconsciousness. Choice (A) is a DNR (Do Not Resuscitate) order. DRG (B) stands for diagnosis-related group.

176. The correct answer is (D).

Res ipsa loquitur means "the thing speaks for itself."

177. The correct answer is (D).

It is the radiographer's responsibility to include on the Introduction of Contrast Material and Radiopharmaceuticals Data Sheet all of the following data: patient allergies, time of administration, and the name of the individual who administers the contrast material.

178. The correct answer is (A).

Nonmaleficence is ethical principles that place high value on avoiding doing harm to others. Fidelity (B) is strict faithfulness and loyalty to others. Morals (C) are generally accepted customs of right and wrong. Autonomy (D) declares that patients are treated as individuals and are to be informed about procedures so that they have the appropriate information to make decisions about their own care.

179. The correct answer is (D).

In an emergency situation, implied consent applies when a patient is unable to give consent because of severe injury. The health care team will operate under the assumption of what the patient would want done if she were conscious and able to give consent.

180. The correct answer is (A).

A deaf patient will rely predominantly on demonstration to communicate with the radiographer. Keep in mind that the deaf patient may also be able to read lips if the radiographer speaks slowly and faces the patient while speaking.

181. The correct answer is (D).

In taking a patient history, good questioning skills would include asking open-ended questions so the patient can elaborate (A), using silence to allow the patient time to remember details (B), and repetition or rewording to clarify information for a more detailed patient history (C).

182. The correct answer is (D).

The effective use of oral communication includes all of the following: giving clear instructions that the patient understands (A), using proper pronunciation (B), and speaking clearly (C).

183. The correct answer is (A).

Hand-washing is a form of medical asepsis. Medical asepsis is the reduction in the number of microorganisms to as few as possible. Hand-washing is the single most important means of preventing the spread of infection.

184. The correct answer is (C).

Autoclaving is the most common method used to sterilize equipment. High temperatures of 275°F to 135°C under high pressure make autoclaving easy and efficient.

185. The correct answer is (B).

Human sweat is the exception. Standard precautions are applied to all patients roomed in isolation. Standard precautions are designed to reduce the transmission of bloodborne and pathogen agents, including blood, mucous membranes, and all body fluids.

186. The correct answer is (D).

The exterior assembly of a urinary tube drainage device must always remain lower than the patient's bladder to prevent the fluid from flowing backwards and causing an infection.

187. The correct answer is (C).

The correct order for opening a sterile pack is as follows: Step 1, the first flap is opened away from the radiographer. Steps 2 and 3, the flaps are opened to the right and the left. Step 4, the last flap is opened toward the radiographer.

188. The correct answer is (D).

When seeing a patient who is in an isolation room and being treated for TB, the radiographer should observe airborne precautions in addition to standard precautions posted. That would include all of the listed special precautions, including the particulate mask worn by the radiographer.

189. The correct answer is (B).

The correct number of room-air changes would be 6 to 12 per hour for an Airborne Precaution isolation room.

190. The correct answer is (A).

Strep throat is a common bacterial infection. AIDS, herpes simplex, and hepatitis are all viruses.

191. The correct answer is (D).

The patient position demonstrated is a Sims' position. Sims' is a semi-oblique prone position, and is the position used for the administration of an enema.

192. The correct answer is (D).

For a two-person lift transfer, the wheelchair should be placed parallel to the table.

193. The correct answer is (B).

On the ECG tracing in the figure shown, the QRS complex represents the contraction of the ventricles.

194. The correct answer is (C).

Dyspnea means shortness of breath. Cyanosis (A) is a bluish discoloration in lips, fingers, and mucus membranes resulting from too little oxygen in the blood. Bradypnea (B) is abnormally slow breathing, and hypoxia (D) means lower-than-normal levels of oxygen in the inspired gases, arterial blood, or tissues.

195. The correct answer is (A).

In an intramuscular injection, the proper needle placement into the muscle is 90°; 45° (B) is for a subcutaneous injection and 15° (D) is for a venipuncture injection.

196. The correct answer is (A).

For an adult patient, a normal BUN blood lab value taken prior to radiographic contrast studies should fall between 7 and 18 mg/dL.

197. The correct answer is (B).

Barium is a positive contrast agent. Air or carbon dioxide would be a negative contrast agent.

198. The correct answer is (A).

Hypotension is a moderate systemic reaction that must be managed appropriately so the patient's condition does not worsen. Mild reactions include metallic taste, urticaria (hives), and vomiting.

199. The correct answer is (B).

The vein identified by Number 1 is the accessory cephalic vein.

200. The correct answer is (C).

The vein identified by Number 4 is the antecubital vein.

How to Assess Your Practice Tests

Taking the full-length practice test in this book can help you simulate the experience of taking the ARRT registry. Each of these contains 200 questions.

The practice test in this book should be taken prior to your first day of study so you can assess yourself. The online practice test should be taken a week or so before the actual exam. For both practice tests, be sure to find a setting in which distractions are minimized, such as a library. Set aside 3.5 hours in total. Taking the exam in such a setting will prepare you for the real testing environment. Avoid any distractions or unnecessary breaks, as these will disrupt your concentration. Remember to bring a calculator and a watch.

After completing the practice test, count the number of questions you answered correctly. While specific information on raw scoring is not available from ARRT, there are some things to keep in mind:

Your test performance is reported as a scaled score—from 1 to 99. (Scaling is a method used to standardize scores and take exam difficulty into account.) To be clear: these are not percentage points; they are scaled scores. Nor are they built on "curves," where a certain percentage would pass and a certain percentage would fail.

A scaled score of **75** is required to pass the exam. In recent years, this has meant approximately 65 percent of answers correct. In other words, out of 200 questions you would need to answer 130 questions correctly to pass. These numbers are not official numbers; they are only a guideline.

Keep in mind that the registry will contain an additional 20 experimental or pilot questions that will not count toward your score.

After you take the online practice test, use it as a final assessment prior to the registry. Ideally, this will serve as a final "tune up" prior to the exam.